THE PARKINSON'S DISEASE HANDBOOK

DR RICHARD GODWIN-AUSTEN is Consultant Neurologist to the Regional Department of Neurology and Neurosurgery in Derby and Nottingham. He was trained at St Thomas's Hospital Medical School and the National Hospital, London, obtained his MD in 1969 and Fellowship of the Royal College of Physicians in 1976. He is a member of the Association of British Neurologists at the Royal College of Physicians, and a Fellow of the Royal Society of Medicine. He has been engaged in clinical research on Parkinson's disease and related subjects since 1968 and has been a member of the medical panel of the Parkinson's Disease Society since 1970. He is married, with two children.

D1248728

Overcoming Common Problems Series

Overcoming Common Problems

THE PARKINSON'S DISEASE HANDBOOK

Dr Richard Godwin-Austen MD, FRCP

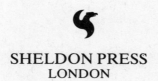

SHELDON PRESS
LONDON

First published in Great Britain in 1984 by
Sheldon Press, SPCK, Marylebone Road, London NW1 4DU

British Library Cataloguing in Publication Data

Godwin Austen, R. B.
  The Parkinson's disease handbook.—(Overcoming
common problems)
  1. Parkinsonism
I. Title   II. Series
616.8′33   RC382
  ISBN 0–85969–411–9
  ISBN 0–85969–397–X pbk

Typeset by Inforum Ltd, Portsmouth
Printed in Great Britain by
Whitstable Litho Ltd, Whitstable, Kent

Contents

Introduction

To be told that you are suffering from Parkinson's disease is, in fact, not always the shattering experience one might suspect. Indeed, many people are relieved to learn that their symptoms are medically recognizable and are not imagined or due to some psychological disorder. There is also the relief that the symptoms do not indicate something more serious – a brain tumour, or premature senility. Inevitably, however, the diagnosis of Parkinson's disease also comes as a great shock. It requires time to accept and adjust to its implications. Most people have heard of Parkinson's disease but their knowledge of the condition usually dates from before modern treatment was available. Gloomy forebodings tend to take the place of the early reassurance that most people are given by their doctor.

It is at this stage that people with Parkinson's disease want to know why it has happened, what they can and should do about it and, above all, what is going to happen to them in the future. Lack of an answer to these questions is perhaps the worst part of being labelled as a sufferer of Parkinson's disease. It is rare nowadays for patients to accept, without question, treatment recommended by a doctor, and most doctors welcome the opportunity to explain and reinforce the effectiveness of their treatment by telling the patient how it works and what the snags and side-effects may be. Many patients derive considerable benefit from becoming an expert on their own medical condition, and with Parkinson's disease it is difficult for anybody else to know as much about the symptoms and response to treatment as the patient himself.

1

This book sets out to explain Parkinson's disease. The aim is to replace the fear of the unknown with an understanding of the disease and its treatment. I have tried to answer all the questions that patients tend to ask, and to give an account of the current medical understanding of what causes the disease, what makes it better or worse, and how the treatment works. It may come as a surprise that so much can be written about one disease, but in a book of this sort the whole range of problems needs to be considered. Nobody must presume that any single individual is going to have to cope with more than a small fraction of the problems described here. All sufferers will recognize some of the problems or symptoms, however, and hopefully will gain reassurance that they are not the only person who has ever suffered in this way.

Armed with the knowledge of what can be done about your condition and what is likely to happen in the future, you will be able to make the best possible plans and arrangements. In this way a positive approach to the disease will allow treatment to achieve its best effect, and avoid the worry and depression that so often obstructs good medical treatment.

The most urgent and immediate question that most patients ask is: 'how rapidly will the disease progress?' This is discussed in detail in the next chapter but in nearly all cases progression is so slow that there is ample time for adjustment. There is, therefore, little real need to be apprehensive about what the future holds. The fact that a diagnosis of Parkinson's disease has been made does not mean that the problems of advancing age are necessarily going to be complicated. And you will be able to plan what adjustments should be made to your home life in good time, and before any major crisis may develop.

After fear of the future, the next major query is whether there is any cure. Parkinson's disease cannot be cured in the way that appendicitis is cured by an operation, but it can be cured in the sense in which diabetes can be cured with insulin. The 'cure', in other words, is relief of symptoms and replacement of deficient chemicals in the brain. But it is dependent on continuing treatment, which must be carefully controlled and adjusted. Like diabetes, Parkinson's disease has complications. It has symptoms that can be only partially overcome and an underlying abnormality that cannot be corrected. We cannot put the clock back to a situation when there was no abnormality any more than we can cure the long-sightedness that afflicts most people in their fifties. An understanding of what the disease is provides the answer to the question of cure, and knowledge of this – as in most conditions – is the only real reassurance.

As we shall see, major research discoveries in the last thirty years have led to dramatic improvements in the treatment of Parkinson's disease. But scientific progress, for all the great benefit it gives, can never substitute for the individual management of the patient. Each patient with this disease is different from every other. Each patient has different physical and mental problems, and has his own home and work surroundings with different family and social relationships.

Perhaps the most important part of treatment of the individual patient is the close supervision by a doctor or specialist who has an interest and knowledge of this disease and its treatment. The relationship between patient and family is also important. The husband or wife, or son or daughter needs to understand the disease, the practical problems it causes and how they can be best overcome. In this way much of the fear of the unknown can be removed. A practical approach can be made to the adaptations necessary to cope with the condition, and everyone can be secure in the knowledge that they are not being deprived of any treatment that might help. The disease doesn't go away. It has to be treated and lived with. But with modern treatment and a positive approach to the problems it poses, most patients find that they can lead a full and enjoyable life.

I would not like to give the impression that all the problems have been solved, however. Parkinson's disease still causes many unpleasant, disabling symptoms which only respond partially or not at all to modern treatment. But the aim of this book is to give the patient and his family a realistic description of what the disease is and how best to avoid or overcome the symptoms. It is important to understand what is going on in the nervous system to cause the disease and how the various treatments work. It is also useful to have this knowledge available in a book, because so often there is insufficient time or opportunity to ask your doctor – and it is helpful and reassuring to be able to turn to the information in such a readily accessible form.

1

What is Parkinson's Disease?

Parkinson's disease, characterized chiefly by tremor and the disturbance of voluntary movement, has probably always afflicted mankind, but was only specifically identified as recently as the last century, and today bears the name of the man who began the serious study of it.

James Parkinson was a family doctor in Shoreditch, in the East End of London, and published his *Essay on the Shaking Palsy* in 1817, when he was sixty-two years old. This short monograph remains one of the classics of medical literature; it includes a description of a patient suffering tremor in a four-poster in a room with Georgian windows where 'the motion becomes so violent as not only to shake the bed-hangings but even the floor and sashes of the room'. Parkinson produced a description of the disease and its evolution during a patient's lifetime so detailed and complete that it scarcely requires any revision today.

Parkinson wrote his essay because he believed that it was important to separate this disease from other causes of tremor and loss of control over movement. Prior to that time patients with any form of paralysis or muscular disorder were considered to be suffering from a 'palsy', and little helpful advice could be given about the likely progression, or otherwise, of their condition or its treatment. The tremor was considered to be the disease, not the symptom. Parkinson emphasized that this particular 'palsy' is neither a paralysis nor a weakness, but rather an extreme slowness of movement,

5

and that this slowness is most severe in the limb most afflicted with the tremor. He was also the first to point out that the disease was distinct from 'the trembling consequent to indulgence in the drinking of spiritous liquors; that which proceeds from the immoderate employment of tea and coffee . . . and that which appears to be dependent upon advanced age'. By describing the disease so accurately, Parkinson laid the foundation upon which subsequent generations of medical specialists have been able to institute treatment.

Medical definition

A person with Parkinson's disease is suffering from disturbances of brain function due to the chemical imbalance of certain nerve cells in one small region of the brain. Different areas of the brain control separate functions of the body – co-ordination, movement, balance and so on – and the proper working of these small areas in the brain depends on a precise balance of chemicals called 'neurotransmitters'. Any disturbance in this chemical balance disturbs the control of co-ordination and movement. In the case of Parkinson's disease the chief chemical abnormality is a deficiency of the 'neurotransmitter' known as dopamine. Exactly what causes this deficiency remains a mystery, and research continues (see Chapter 9).

Parkinson's disease is known as a 'degenerative' disease. This means that it results from a failure of a bodily function rather than an inflammation or the growth of abnormal tissue – which is what causes cancer, for example. The area of the brain which degenerates in Parkinson's disease is a group of concentrations of nerve cells near the base of the brain; some of these are unusual in being pigmented – black – and are consequently called the 'substantia nigra' or 'black substance'. In normal circumstances these cells generate practically all the dopamine in the brain. When dopamine is not synthesized by these cells there is a failure of that part of the brain to function normally which causes the symptoms of Parkinson's disease. If the chemical balance is redressed, the disease can be abated (see Chapter 4).

Parkinson's disease therefore results from the gradual and progressive loss of nerve cells in the substantia nigra. The cell loss is extremely slow, and for years surviving cells compensate for the loss of function; it is probably not until nearly half the cells have degenerated that the first symptoms of the disease appear. Then, perhaps as the result of some added stress or fatigue, the compensatory mechanisms are no longer adequate and the first symptoms emerge – often to disappear again when calmer circumstances prevail. But sooner or later continuous symptoms become obvious. The disease continues to progress, but the rate of progression varies enormously between different individuals. Before the days of effective treatment it was evident that some patients deteriorated so rapidly that their disease deprived them of their independence within three or four years of the time of diagnosis. In others, more than twenty years could pass before the disease had progressed to this point. Nowadays the progressive nature of Parkinson's disease may be entirely concealed by effective treatment.

Myths

Now that the medical origins of Parkinson's disease have been identified, it is possible to dismiss all the rumours, fallacies and old wives' tales that have built up around people suffering from tremor. As with many diseases, these stories cause unnecessary distress and may even be a definite hindrance to dealing with the disease.

Most patients come to the doctor with their own idea as to the cause of the disease. Many blame some traumatic experience, or perhaps some injury or illness. A surgical operation may seem to have marked the onset of symptoms. There is no medical evidence that factors such as these cause the disease, although it is possible that they provide a trigger in some cases.

Still at home, some patients remember a relative who suffered from Parkinson's disease, and begin to wonder whether there is an inherited weakness which makes them susceptible. This possibility has been carefully investigated in many extensive surveys, and it is now clear that the chances of the disease being inherited are almost negligible. The best test of this is to study identical twins who, having an identical genetic make-up, should both develop any disease that is caused by an inherited defect. In one recent study, thirty-seven sufferers of Parkinson's disease were located who were also identical twins; significantly, only two of their twins had also developed the disease, an incidence no greater than would be expected in any random group of such a size. This effectively excludes any element of inheritance.

Surprisingly, some patients still believe the old stories about eating and drinking leading to the disease. Diet, either over-indulgence or deficiency of some vital element, has not been discovered to have any bearing on Parkinson's disease. Certainly, over-indulgence in alcohol, tobacco, tea or coffee (all popular culprits before Parkinson) is not a cause of the disease; indeed, it appears that smokers are significantly *less* likely to develop the disease than non-smokers (although once the disease has developed, smoking is of no benefit). It also seems that being overweight or underweight has no bearing on parkinsonism.

The increasing incidence of the disease, which is probably due to increasing longevity, has led to speculation that overwork and stress can lead to developing Parkinson's disease. This, too, can be dismissed, as can the other extreme, laziness. When the disease develops doctors do not tell the patient to ease up, let alone stop work – in fact, the general rule is to keep going, as will be emphasized later.

Stages of the disease

Doctors find it useful to distinguish between various stages of the disease as it allows them to recommend different types of treatment at a time when they are most likely to be beneficial.

In the early stages of the disease there are symptoms which are a nuisance, but constitute no disability or handicap: tremor which causes embarrassment, or an awkwardness with fine movement which makes certain tasks slow and laborious. As the disease gets worse a stage is reached where the symptoms produce a definite disability, so that certain tasks have to be avoided altogether, or can only be done at certain times of the day. The disease may therefore limit the length of time that the sufferer can spend gardening or writing before fatigue and slowness of movement compels them to do something else. This is the 'major symptomatic' stage, where the untreated disease limits activity but does not deprive the patient of independence.

Further progression of the disease results in a late stage where the patient is no longer able to do everything for himself. Independence may be increasingly lost, as help is required with bathing, dressing, shaving and washing, and even cutting up food.

With modern treatment the life expectancy of a patient with Parkinson's disease is little different from that of the rest of the population. Nevertheless, Parkinson's disease, in advanced cases, causes complications which may prove fatal. Pneumonia, kidney failure, weight loss, and blood infections may overwhelm the patient debilitated by the disease. But it should be emphasized that this is not a painful disease: as one patient once remarked to me, with considerable doubt in his voice, 'I suppose . . . *most* of us have to die of something . . . eventually.'

Related diseases

Before leaving the definition of the disease, we must consider briefly some rare 'sub-groups' of parkinsonism.

Perhaps the commonest cause of symptoms resembling those of Parkinson's disease are the side-effects of drugs. In particular, a group of tranquillizers called phenothiazines will, if given in high enough doses, cause symptoms closely resembling those of Parkinson's disease and referred to as 'parkinsonism'. When the drug is stopped the patient recovers, but there are some in whom continuing treatment with these drugs is essential for their mental health. To some extent the secondary parkinsonism which they develop can be relieved by the same treatment given to sufferers of Parkinson's disease.

Between 1917 and 1927 an apparently new disease appeared called *Encephalitis lethargica* – a very serious and frequently fatal brain fever. Among those who did survive the disease, there was a very high incidence of a form of parkinsonism. This type of the disease, known as 'post-encephalitic parkinsonism', is often non-progressive, and may be associated with other psychological or neurological disabilities. It may not appear until years after the original brain fever. *Encephalitis lethargica* has been extremely rare since about 1927, so that the incidence of this form of parkinsonism has diminished and continues to do so. The response to treatment of patients is different to those with Parkinson's disease, so they should be treated by a neurologist who has particular knowledge of the disease.

Finally, there are a number of neurological diseases in which parkinsonism develops as a part of the disease. In general, any condition that affects the normal activity in the substantia nigra or nearby areas of the brain may give rise to parkinsonism. Occasionally, therefore, brain tumours or strokes may imitate Parkinson's disease, or other degenerative processes may result in parkinsonian symptoms. The distinction between Parkinson's disease and these conditions is vitally important, because treatment must obviously be directed to the underlying cause of the parkinsonian symptoms. Treatment with drugs for Parkinson's disease may merely cover up the illness without obtaining a cure. Furthermore, the diagnosis of secondary parkinsonism may be very difficult. The opinion of a neurologist is usually advisable wherever there is any doubt.

11

2

Living with the Major Symptoms

The symptom most commonly associated with Parkinson's disease is tremor, although in fact nearly half the patients with the disease have no tremor when the first symptoms develop. Nevertheless, tremor remains the most characteristic and obvious symptom of the majority of patients sooner or later. It is usually complicated by the two other cardinal symptoms of Parkinson's disease – stiffness of the muscles and slowness of movement. These three symptoms will be discussed in detail in this chapter, together with the other symptoms commonly associated with them. Less common features of the disease are discussed in Chapter 3.

In this description of the symptoms of Parkinson's disease I have aimed at being comprehensive; however, some of them are actually quite rare. So do not expect to develop all or even most of these symptoms! On the other hand, you may develop symptoms that are not mentioned but are nevertheless due to Parkinson's disease.

Tremor

The tremor caused by Parkinson's disease is so distinctive that it is surprising how often it is confused with the tremors brought about by other causes. This confusion has led to a number of people being unnecessarily treated for Parkinson's disease. The tremor most often confused with Parkinson's disease is that known as 'benign essential tremor', seen so commonly in the elderly. This is not due to any disease but may be inherited or caused by anxiety.

Parkinsonian tremor is typically one-sided, and most often obvious in only one hand or arm. It is usually present when the patient is at rest, especially when nervous or particularly tired. It may also appear only when the arm is held in a certain position. Some patients find that they can suppress the tremor by holding the arm bent or, perhaps surprisingly, by carrying something in the affected hand. The tremor is quite slow – about four or six beats per second, compared with the twelve beats per second of a normal shiver.

Perhaps the most important characteristic of parkinsonian tremor is that it disappears during sleep and decreases in severity, or may disappear altogether, when the affected limb is used. This often means that the tremor itself causes relatively little disability; a shaking hand can become still and controllable enough for a cup of tea or a glass of water to be lifted without spilling a drop.

Any tremor, however severe in itself, however, can be troublesome because it attracts attention, and is difficult to conceal. The more you try to prevent people noticing, the more the nervous tension and embarrassment make the tremor difficult to control. This reaction often discourages people suffering from Parkinson's disease from enjoying their social life to the full, especially meeting new people, and from potentially awkward situations like eating in a restaurant. In this case, a tremor which is in itself less physically disabling than some other symptoms can end up causing more disruption to the patient's life than anything else associated with the disease.

So how does one deal with tremor? To begin with, it is essential to understand that tremor is a symptom which it is difficult to suppress completely by medical treatment. So do not expect to get rid of it altogether, and above all do not sit back and wait for the treatment to work. It all boils down to a question of learning to live with it, and to developing a new attitude. If you can ignore it, you will find that other people do the same. Of course, there are times when a tremor is bound to distract people, but the right approach will usually make things easier. A patient of mine was required as part of his job to give a number of lectures. Far from trying to conceal his tremor, he would accustom his audience to it by making a few light-hearted references to it early on. He would then put his hand behind his back or in his pocket, and invariably found that his audience forgot all about it from then on.

While tremor is worse as a result of nervousness, it is *not caused* by nervousness or stress, but by the rhythmical electrical discharge of malfunctioning nerve cells in the brain described in the last chapter. This points the way to a more complex way of dealing with it. The transmission of tremor is through a specific and very localized region of the brain, and a surgical operation to destroy this region and relieve tremor is still occasionally carried out – although much less commonly than it was before the days of effective medical treatment. Any brain operation is clearly an alarming prospect, but nowadays the operation is only performed where the risks are minimal and the benefits cannot be achieved by any other means of treatment. A fine needle is used to freeze (literally) the area of brain tissue which produces the tremor, which is only 3mm across. In suitable cases the technique is marvellously successful. In the majority, however, a combination of drug treatments will so improve tremor that surgery is not required, and there is never any sense in running the small but inevitable risks of surgery if these can be avoided.

Rigidity

Most people with Parkinson's disease are unaware initially of any stiffness or rigidity of their muscles, and this feature of the disease is often only revealed after a doctor's examination helps to confirm the overall diagnosis. But muscular stiffness does cause a number of important symptoms which are commonplace and cause many patients considerable distress. The most important of these is pain.

Pain is a symptom of so many arthritic and muscular conditions that the patient who complains of pain which is caused by Parkinson's disease may be misdiagnosed as suffering from a slipped disc or similar condition. Treatment for these conditions will not relieve the painful rigidity from the Parkinson's disease, and effective parkinsonian treatment is, of course, what is required.

The pain caused by Parkinson's disease is most commonly felt in the neck, shoulders and arms; the back or leg muscles may also be affected. It is a continuous aching discomfort, which is made worse by muscular exercise or fatigue. Usually pain is associated with a general feeling of exhaustion, and a disinclination to leave the favourite chair, but even when sitting still the aching remains troublesome and unrelieved by ordinary pain-killing tablets.

Pain from Parkinson's disease may sometimes be

15

THE PARKINSON'S DISEASE HANDBOOK

localized in the upper part of the neck or head, and the patient may suspect they have a brain tumour – especially if they notice a difficulty in moving one side of the body. In other cases chest pain may suggest a heart condition so that there is an understandable sense of relief when the correct diagnosis is made.

Rigidity of muscles may produce an apparent weakness – for example weakness of grip or in lifting an arm. In fact, when muscular strength is tested it can be shown to be normal, and the patient is really complaining of the rigidity hampering the normal freedom of movement. Rigidity of the muscles is nearly always associated with the third and most characteristic symptom of Parkinson's disease: slowness of movement.

Slowness of movement

There are many manifestations of 'hypokinesia' (which is the medical term for slowness of movement). It affects everyday movements such as walking, getting out of a chair or turning over in bed. Speech, swallowing and facial expression may also be involved, and slowness of movement in the arms affects writing and other movements of the hands.

To the patient, slowness of movement is a difficult symptom to describe, or understand. Many patients attribute it to 'old age', and unfortunately the doctor may sometimes accept this explanation, unfortunate because, unlike the aches of old age, this slowness can usually be relieved by treatment. Many people also put down their slowness of movement to psychological causes.

Hypokinesia is the most important feature in the

diagnosis of Parkinson's disease and nearly always the most disabling. It produces the typical expressionless face which so often is mistaken for stupidity or loss of intelligence – quite wrongly, as will be explained in the next chapter. It leads to a lack of natural movements, such as blinking or swinging the arms when walking. Even when nervous, the Parkinson's disease patient does not fidget but sits quite still, failing to turn his head or move his hands.

The disability from hypokinesia arises from the fact that all voluntary movements become slow, reduced in range and require considerably more effort and concentration to achieve. Thus, walking becomes slower and the length of each individual pace is shortened. When the disease affects one side of the body more than the other, the affected leg may drag, and the toe of the shoe catch on pavements or carpets.

Repetitive movements of the arm are particularly difficult – stirring a saucepan, polishing, brushing teeth or working up a lather for shaving are all mammoth tasks. Characteristically, writing also becomes slow, spidery and untidy, and tends to get smaller the longer it is continued in one session. In some cases writing will come to an involuntary halt, and require a specific effort of will to resume. Other fine movements of the fingers are also affected: changing an electric plug, using a screwdriver, for example, or more commonplace, turning the page of a book, doing cuff or shirt buttons, bra hooks, or cutting up food. Where one hand is especially affected, it makes two-handed tasks difficult because the good hand wants to go faster than the bad one; peeling potatoes or tying shoelaces are good examples.

Hypokinesia is disturbing because it involves more

17

than what we normally consider as movement. Slowness of speech and the inability to raise the voice is a symptom which is particularly troublesome for people doing jobs such as teaching or lecturing. Parkinsonian slowness of movement affects the muscles of the chest and diaphragm as well as those of the larynx, and as a result speech becomes softer, slower and slightly slurred. By a sudden effort of will it is usually possible for the patient to shout out a loud single word or phrase, even when otherwise speech is very soft; frustratingly, this variability may only lead relatives to suspect that the complaint is 'psychological', that the patient is imagining the difficulty or putting it on. When the speech problems become obvious under circumstances of stress, such as speaking in public, such an explanation seems attractive; it is not, however, correct, and it follows that even a sustained effort of will cannot significantly overcome the problem.

Relatives and friends may find the slowness of movement irritating and frustrating, but it is characteristic of Parkinson's disease that however much he may try the patient cannot hurry. Tasks such as dressing, washing and feeding take much longer than they used to, and it becomes important to make allowances for this. The patient, of course, finds the slowness of movement more frustrating than anyone, because his mind is moving much faster than his muscles, and he is far more exasperated than anyone else at how slowly he performs simple tasks.

This last fact emphasizes that the slowness is confined to movement. Mental agility and the speed of thought processes are retained, the only exceptions being in the more advanced cases or where side-effects of treatment play a part. But the general rule is that

Parkinson's disease does not lead to any slowing up in the mind at all. This must be recognised by relatives, since there is nothing more distressing than to be treated as an imbecile when your only difficulties are physical.

Disturbance of balance

Slowness of movement is an important part of the symptom of dizziness or disturbance of balance which is so common in patients with Parkinson's disease. Most people notice difficulty when getting out of a low chair. They are frightened of falling forwards and as a result seldom place their feet far enough under the chair to make it easy to stand up.

This is only one aspect of disturbance of balance, however. When standing or moving about the house, turning round may be difficult because the feet seem 'stuck to the floor'. A similar difficulty may arise when you try to walk – in an effort to overcome the resistance to movement, balance is lost, the legs give way, and a fall results. Some patients have particular difficulty at the threshold of a door, where for some inexplicable reason the feet seem to 'dither' and not want to move. . . In this situation, too, balance may go. Walking down an incline is especially difficult. The legs feel as if they are going to 'run away with you', and indeed may occasionally do so. Many patients find it necessary to have support and assistance when walking downhill, even though when on level ground their balance is good. Climbing on a bus or train is difficult and slow, and if the bus goes off before you have sat down loss of balance is almost inevitable. In crowds there is a particular problem, because any tendency to be bumped may throw the person with Parkinson's disease off balance and cause them to fall. This will be discussed in detail in the next chapter, but slowness of movement prevents the parkinsonian sufferer from recovering balance.

There are certain bodily movements that seem to be particularly affected in Parkinson's disease. Turning over in bed has already been mentioned, and ways of coping with this difficulty will be discussed in Chapter 5. But getting in or out of a car – never an easy manoeuvre even for the able-bodied – is particularly difficult for the parkinsonian. The bath poses similar problems. It is not just the slowness and awkwardness of movement but the fear of falling which increasingly limits activity. It becomes a vicious circle if confidence cannot be regained by treatment or adaptations to daily living. The patient who is frightened of injuring himself in a fall tends to spend more and more time in a chair, and avoids getting out and about. As the result he cannot obtain the exercise which is so necessary for maintaining mobility and relieving the stiffness of the muscles (see Chapter 5). Furthermore, medical treatment is only effective when it is used by the patient to enable him to become active. Loss of confidence and fear of falling may therefore lead to a depressed state of mind which requires great courage and insight to escape from.

3

Minor Symptoms

Tremor, rigidity and slowness of movement have always been considered the major and most important symptoms of Parkinson's disease. But some patients would not agree with this assessment. To many, indeed, symptoms such as tiredness, depression, dribbling, constipation or mental confusion cause the major difficulties, and it is these and similar matters which will be discussed in this chapter.

The roll-call of these minor symptoms can seem endless. There is sometimes difficulty in deciding whether or not a symptom is due to Parkinson's disease at all. Certainly, it is not possible to mention every symptom that may be due to Parkinson's disease in a book of this length. If you have a complaint that is not mentioned here, I would recommend you to seek medical advice. Further treatment or investigation may be necessary; alternatively, it may be all part of Parkinson's disease, and possible to deal with by suitable changes in treatment.

In any patient who has been diagnosed, there is a substantial incidence of side-effects from the first parkinsonian treatment. These may give rise to symptoms difficult to distinguish from symptoms of the disease. These side-effects of the treatment are discussed in the chapter on treatment (Chapter 4), so if there is some complaint which is not mentioned in this chapter, and you are on treatment, look it up there.

Tiredness

Most of us believe, rather self-indulgently, that we suffer from excessive tiredness from time to time. Most people do not know real tiredness, but it is a common feature of Parkinson's disease. It is difficult to describe, and as difficult to understand if you do not have the disease. Patients with Parkinson's disease have to make a very great effort to achieve what, to any normal person, would be ordinary physical exercise. After working in the garden for half an hour, a sense of complete exhaustion may be felt and, what is worse, rest does not seem to relieve the exhaustion in the way it should.

The tiredness is not only a physical thing – it is mental as well. There is a lethargy and disinclination to develop interests which is part of the disease. This symptom has to be understood by both patient and family so that as far as possible steps can be taken to overcome it. In this way a positive effort can be made to develop social activities, continue interests and take regular exercise. Initially any increase of activity in this way may scarcely seem worth the draining effort it demands, but in the long run it is hard to think of any part of the treatment which is more important.

Sleep

The need for a satisfactory night's sleep is increased in any case of Parkinson's disease. Most patients need a full eight or nine hours sleep at night, and some benefit from an extra snooze of up to an hour after lunch or in the evening. What must be avoided is 'nodding off' in the chair, either morning, noon or evening. This will only lead to unsatisfactory quality of sleep at night, with the attendant complications of confusion and hallucinations. A good night's sleep will often have a remarkable effect on the other symptoms of Parkinson's disease. Although sedative drugs may be necessary, the best way of ensuring satisfactory sleep is to have been sufficiently active during the day.

Depression

This is so common that it is almost a constant feature of Parkinson's disease. In the early stages of the disease there is a vague feeling of nervous irritability as if 'things aren't quite right'. In some patients severe symptoms of depression develop, with feelings of guilt, weepiness, lack of energy and even suicidal thoughts. Much time is taken up with worrying about the disease, about specific symptoms and other matters which can't be put right by worry. Depression often leads to early waking so that the dawn is spent lying awake ruminating on all the troubles, and so things worsen.

Such a reaction is not caused by horror at the diagnosis, but is part of the disease. Indeed, even though the physical response to treatment is good, the mental condition often deteriorates when treatment is started. Specific treatment for depression is therefore usually required, and it is important to draw your doctor's attention to symptoms of depression so that he can recommend suitable measures. This is especially important – people with depression often do not seek medical advice, because they feel that it is all their own fault and that they only need to 'pull themselves together'. This is seldom, if ever, true; on the contrary, symptoms of the type described nearly always have a medical cause and, most importantly, can be treated effectively.

Memory

We would all like to have better memories and if there was a drug that would improve our memory it would sell like hot cakes. But there are many people with Parkinson's disease who have a significant impairment in memory. This is very seldom bad enough to cause handicap, however, and is usually merely a matter of making adjustments so that a lapse of memory does not lead to difficulties. At work or at home a notepad becomes essential, and lists of appointments and shopping needs smooth over the problem.

An unusual and characteristic symptom related to impairment of memory is 'thought block'. In the course of conversation the patient with Parkinson's disease may suddenly come to a complete halt and be unable to remember what he was saying. There is an embarrassed silence while he struggles to remember what the conversation was about, and then it all comes back and he can continue normally. Thought block is a worrying symptom – I have had patients who thought they were going mad. But in fact it is not a serious symptom from a medical standpoint. It does not indicate any progressive mental deterioration or psychological abnormality. Unfortunately it is not amenable to any treatment currently available, but it is important to note that thought block may, in some cases, be made worse by the group of drugs called the anticholinergics.

More difficulties with walking

There are a number of very specific and often rather bizarre symptoms that are not strictly ascribable to slowness of movement, but which affect walking. The commonest of these is 'start hesitancy'.

When a patient with Parkinson's disease wants to step off to walk, he may find that he is unable to do so because the automatic movement of lifting one foot off the ground and moving it forward is prevented. The reason for this seems to be that Parkinson's disease makes it difficult to induce the reflex reaction to shift the centre of gravity on to the one foot so that the other can be lifted and moved forward. The symptom is often variable, so that some times of the day there may be no difficulty whereas at others walking at all becomes almost impossible. This variability may lead relatives and friends to be unsympathetic and suspect that you are not trying – but, on the contrary, the harder you try the greater the difficulty becomes. The difficulty in lengthening the stride has already been mentioned, but it is interesting to find that many patients have much less difficulty moving their legs when climbing stairs than when they are on the flat.

In some cases, if a patient is given a small push from behind or in front, they will topple and then start to walk with little paces chasing their centre of gravity. Out of control, they are unable to stop until they either fall or come up against a wall or other obstruction. This is a frightening and embarrassing symptom, and one which is horribly hard to understand. It is called retropulsion or propulsion, and it is a particular danger in crowded places. I often recommend that patients with this symptom should always carry a stick, thereby

25

drawing attention to the fact that they have some difficulty with walking, and making it less likely that people will bump into them. The added support that a stick gives may also go a long way to preventing the symptom.

Posture

The characteristic posture of the sufferer of Parkinson's disease is slightly stooped, with rounded shoulders and the arms and legs bent at elbows, hips and knees. This posture places added strain on the joints and muscles of the back and neck, and may be partly the cause of pain.

When sitting, patients with disease affecting one side more than the other may lean to one side, so that they need a chair with an arm on that side for support. When walking, there is often the tendency to hold one arm bent across the trunk instead of swinging normally by the side.

All these disturbances of posture are correctable voluntarily, but tend to relapse as soon as the effort to adopt a normal posture is inevitably forgotten. Many patients are unaware of any abnormality of posture until it is pointed out to them or they notice it in the mirror long after it has been obvious to others. It is certainly a minor inconvenience at times, but never a serious symptom.

Dribbling

One of the most distressing and socially disabling symptoms is dribbling. This is not due to any excess of saliva, although the most frequently recommended treatment is with drugs to dry the mouth.

26

Parkinson's disease reduces the frequency of the automatic movement of swallowing, which normally gets rid of the flow of saliva. In addition, the disturbance of posture described above means that the head is sometimes held tilted forwards, so that saliva tends to accumulate in the front of the mouth. It is important, therefore, to try to adopt a sitting posture that encourages the head to tilt backwards. Useful measures include a pillow in the back with a chair that slopes backwards and is not too upright, and the placing of any television set high enough to be seen looking slightly upwards.

Swallowing is another difficulty associated with dribbling, but any such difficulty is often due to a complicated combination of factors. Not only does the disease itself, in some cases, result in difficulty in swallowing, but also the drugs may make it worse by causing dryness of the mouth or spasm of muscles in the throat. If symptoms of this type develop you should ask your doctor's advice. There may be the need for more or different treatment. In general, food of a soft consistency is the easiest to swallow, and it is wise to avoid dry lumpy foods on the one hand, and sharp or excessively sweet liquids on the other.

Constipation

In Parkinson's disease the normal muscular activity of the bowel is reduced. Constipation is therefore extremely common in patients with this condition, and it is often made worse by anticholinergic drugs. In any case, reduced physical exercise and activity tend to lead to constipation. The treatment of constipation is considered in detail in Chapter 6.

Do not let this symptom become an obsession. It rarely causes major problems or difficulties whereas the excessive use of laxatives can lead to major problems – even incontinence – and it is quite unnecessary to spend a lot of time worrying about constipation. A bowel movement about three times a week is perfectly satisfactory.

Eyesight

It is not uncommon to have difficulty in focusing on nearby objects because the parkinsonian may lose the ability to converge with the eyes in order to focus. This leads to blurring of vision, often with double vision when reading. Relief can often be obtained by incorporating a slight prismatic correction in the prescription for reading glasses.

Focusing movement of the eyes may be slowed in Parkinson's disease, a particular problem when driving, where you may find that you are unable to shift gaze quickly. This symptom usually improves with treatment but, if not, obviously constitutes a reason for giving up driving.

The reduction in frequency of blinking may lead to a dryness of the eyes, and a tendency to crusting of the eyelids and soreness of the eyes. Artificial tears (Hypromellose drops) instilled into the eyes with a dropper several times a day may be extremely helpful.

Finally, the anticholinergic drugs often used to treat Parkinson's disease may affect focusing, and it is usual when patients are first put on these drugs to notice that near vision is slightly blurred. It is best not to rush off and change your reading glasses – visual response often improves with continuing treatment, and no change

28

may be necessary. Very occasionally anticholinergic drugs cause a rise in the fluid pressure in the eye and provoke glaucoma, which is a condition of raised pressure in the eye causing pain, vomiting and deterioration of vision. They should never, therefore, be taken by anyone with a history of glaucoma and any pain or severe deterioration of vision while taking these drugs should be reported immediately to the doctor.

Skin problems

Characteristically, Parkinson's disease leads to a rather greasy, scaly skin. This condition is called seborrhoea, and results in greasy hair and eyebrows with irritation and dandruff, and a rather greasy, shiny complexion. Interestingly, drugs whose action is on the brain, such as those used in treating Parkinson's disease, tend to improve these disturbances of the skin. In addition, frequent and regular shampooing of the hair, especially with shampoos containing selenium sulphide (ask for these at your chemist), and washing the skin daily with normal soap, are useful in keeping the problem under control.

In some patients, excessive sweating is a problem. This may be particularly troublesome at night. Its cause is unknown but, as a symptom, it is more common in post-encephalitic cases (see Chapter 1). It usually responds well to standard parkinsonian treatment with anticholinergic drugs but occasionally additional medical treatment has to be used.

Swelling of the ankles

As many of us know, swelling of the feet and ankles develops if we have to sit still for long periods of time, on a long journey for example. This is because the circulation in the legs is dependent on the pumping action of the muscles of the calf and thighs. Patients with Parkinson's disease who may be unable to move their legs normally, and who anyway tend to remain seated for long periods without the normal restless shuffling of their feet, may develop swelling of the ankles. This symptom is likely to be particularly severe in hot weather, and it may be made worse by some forms of treatment. Ankle swelling may even become bad enough to cause difficulty in wearing normal shoes, and there is a risk of skin complications or phlebitis.

Treatment should be aimed at improving blood circulation. When sitting, put your feet up, ideally to waist level, on the arm of a sofa or a high footstool. Elastic stockings put on first thing in the morning may be very helpful for men as well as women. Once again, regular exercise with walking is beneficial – even wriggling the toes and up-down movements of the ankle are useful.

Unrelated minor symptoms

Of course, having Parkinson's disease does not protect you from other illnesses or the symptoms that they cause. Since Parkinson's disease usually develops in the second half of life, there may be other conditions causing the symptoms which you may be tempted to blame on the Parkinson's disease or its treatment. Arthritis of the hip, for example, may make walking

30

much more difficult, but what is required is pain-killing treatment or an operation, not parkinsonian treatment. Arthritis of other joints similarly may need treatment with painkillers, physiotherapy or heat.

Shortness of breath may prevent exercise and activity, and thereby reduce the effectiveness of parkinsonian treatment. Shortness of breath is unlikely to be due to Parkinson's disease, but probably indicates a heart or lung disorder which may need treatment in its own right.

Prostate enlargement in men may give rise to slowness in passing water. Anticholinergic drugs and constipation tend to make this problem worse, and surgical treatment of the enlarged prostate gland may become necessary. Finally, failing vision and memory in the elderly are of course commonplace, and cannot be blamed on Parkinson's disease.

Summary

This chapter has reviewed a large number of symptoms, many of them relatively trivial in themselves, which may combine to constitute severe disability. Most of them can be helped by treatment or adjustments to life style, and these matters will be considered in greater detail later.

It is important to repeat that you should not expect to develop all or even most of the symptoms described. Many of them are rare and most patients only recognize a very few of these symptoms as part of their experience of Parkinson's disease.

31

4

Medical Treatment

Treatment of Parkinson's disease by drugs has a history of only about a century, and today there are two main groups of drugs, both of which have been developed even more recently, since the last war. The advances in treatment which have been introduced in the last twenty years have produced enormous benefit for patients with this condition.

After James Parkinson's specific identification of the disease in 1817, it was not until the 1880s that neurologists in Paris discovered that drugs derived from the belladonna group of plants led to some relief in rigidity and tremor. These simple drugs were the main treatment until the 1940s, when they were superseded by chemically synthesized and concentrated agents which worked in the same way. This group, known as the anticholinergics, meant that for the first time drug treatment for Parkinson's disease was widely available. These drugs are still in use today, but their role in treatment has been reduced by the introduction of much more effective drugs called the dopaminergics which replace the most important chemical deficient in the brain in Parkinson's disease.

It was in Sweden in the 1960s that the role of the chemical dopamine as a messenger within the brain (described in Chapter 1) was first suggested. Soon afterwards, scientists in Vienna identified Parkinson's disease with a deficiency in dopamine, and this has led to the use of levodopa, which is the natural chemical precursor of dopamine, as a treatment to replace the deficiency. Levodopa, therefore, was the first dopaminergic or dopamine-active drug to be shown to be effective in treatment. Subsequently synthetic agents with a similar action have been produced – drugs like bromocriptine or pergolide, which will be discussed later.

Inevitably, with these improvements in treatment, side-effects and complications have arisen. These drugs are not easy to use and every patient with Parkinson's disease presents a different combination of problems and therefore a different response to treatment. Great care is necessary to be certain to achieve the maximum benefit in each individual case. Furthermore, treatment is in most cases going to be necessary over many years, and frequently decades. The response to treatment also alters with the passage of time, and as the disease gets worse. It therefore becomes important to use a combination of treatments which gives the greatest advantage in the short-term combined with the minimum incidence of side-effects in the long-term, as such side-effects frequently result in the dose of effective treatment having to be reduced.

Prescription of drugs

The aim of drug treatment for Parkinson's disease is to keep the patient active, independent and free of handicap. However, it is not necessarily in the patient's best interests to raise the dose of drugs to the point where symptoms disappear completely, because this may necessitate such high dosage that side-effects are provoked.

The compromise necessary is usually reflected in the treatment prescribed. Treatment with drugs containing levodopa tends to restore the concentration of dopamine towards normal and thereby alleviates the symptoms. But, with the development of Parkinson's disease, some brain cells containing a substance called acetyl choline react to the lack of dopamine by increasing activity. Far from improving the symptoms this reaction makes them worse. Treatment with anticholinergic drugs damps down this excessive nerve cell activity and leads to further improvement in symptoms. The two groups of drugs, dopaminergic and anticholinergic, therefore act as if they are at opposite ends of a see-saw – tending to tilt it towards the normal and away from the parkinsonian state.

The benefits of levodopa-containing drugs and anticholinergic preparation therefore add up, and the one group of drugs is complementary to the other. It is fortunate that the side-effects of each of these two groups of drugs do not 'add up' in the same way. Normally it is best for most patients to be maintained on some drugs from each group, even though this tends to make treatment somewhat complicated. It is important to realize that because you may be prescribed more than one drug, it does not mean that your condition is more severe. Indeed, as we shall see later, additional treatment may be required for specific symptoms, sometimes adding up to four or five different preparations.

Patients are often frightened by the large number of tablets that they are taking and have visions of these either reacting with each other in the body or accumulating in the system. Neither of these fears is realistic – the drugs that are used for Parkinson's disease and its secondary symptoms do not inter-react, except in very rare and well-recognized instances. These are well known to doctors and such drug combinations are easily avoided. Nearly all the drugs used are broken down and destroyed in the body within twenty-four hours, so that there is no risk of accumulation. The change in response to a drug that may be noticeable with the passage of time is not due to accumulation of the drug in the body. The nervous system tends to alter its response to these drugs and in general to become more sensitive to them with long exposure, and it is this increasing sensitivity that leads to any change in response.

In the treatment of many medical conditions treatment is standardized, but in Parkinson's disease the drugs used, the timing and the size of the doses have to be adjusted according to the severity and type of symptom from which the patient is suffering. Generally speaking, the early, young or mild case requires treatment only with small doses of anticholinergic drugs, often with the addition of a drug such as amantadine (see later). There may also be the need for antidepressant drugs or treatment for constipation or pain; and tremor may also require specific treatment.

The more severe case, in which symptoms are causing increasing handicap, requires the introduction of a levodopa drug (such as Madopar or Sinemet) and it is usual at this stage to withdraw amantadine. If the symptoms increase, the dose of levodopa has to be increased – up to the maximum tolerated. At this stage, it may be necessary to introduce additional treatment with other dopaminergic drugs such as bromocriptine or pergolide. Additional treatment may be necessary if there are symptoms such as pain, sleeplessness or confusion which cannot be controlled by the other drugs. It is now time to examine the mode of action, benefits and side-effects of each of the major drugs used in the treatment of Parkinson's disease.

Levodopa

The overall improvement which may be expected by using a levodopa drug, about seventy per cent, is substantially greater than that which can be achieved by any other drug currently available. On the other side of the balance, however, one must consider the inevitable short and long-term side-effects.

As has been explained, levodopa is the substance from which the body manufactures dopamine, the chemical whose deficiency, in certain brain cells, causes Parkinson's disease. Levodopa is used because dopamine itself cannot be absorbed by mouth, and would have to be given by injection.

The levodopa is absorbed from the intestine and carried via the liver by the bloodstream to the brain. The conversion to dopamine involves an enzyme or protein called decarboxylase, which unfortunately occurs widely throughout the body. Left to its own devices, therefore, the body would convert all the levodopa into dopamine well before it reached the brain, which is where it is really needed. Levodopa drugs therefore also contain a decarboxylase inhibitor, a harmless chemical which keeps the levodopa intact until it reaches the brain, but importantly, does not enter the brain, remaining instead in the bloodstream (Fig.1). If the decarboxylase inhibitor entered the brain it would prevent levodopa being converted to dopamine where it is needed – in the brain.

All the symptoms of Parkinson's disease tend to be improved by levodopa treatment, but it is most

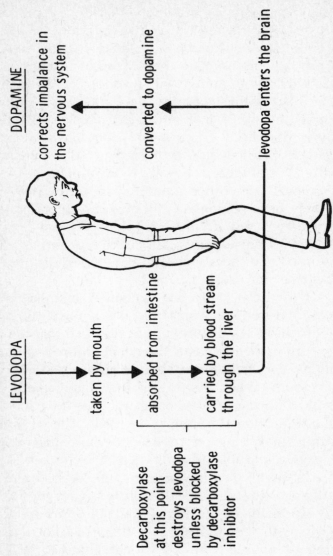

Figure 1

effective of all in relieving slowness of movement and related symptoms. It is no exaggeration to say that improvement can be dramatic when levodopa treatment is started. When it was first introduced, patients who had been bed-ridden for years were able to walk and use their limbs again. Now it is not uncommon to see a patient on treatment with levodopa in whom there are no detectable features of Parkinson's disease, because the drug has alleviated the characteristic posture, impaired facial expression and associated movement difficulties. Rigidity and pain are also usually substantially relieved by levodopa.

Tremor, on the other hand, may in some cases show relatively little response – although in others marked improvement may occur. The symptoms that respond least well to levodopa treatment are disturbances of swallowing and speech and (in some cases) disturbance of balance and 'start hesitancy'.

Unfortunately, there are a number of minor side-effects of levodopa which may be noticed. In some patients there is a disturbance of taste, so that tea and coffee in particular taste 'metallic'. More generally, many patients find that the drug causes a nasty taste in their mouth. When the drug is first taken, there may also be disturbance of sleep, if the last dose is taken within four hours of going to bed. There is then difficulty in getting off to sleep because the mind is over-active and unable to 'switch off'. Some patients notice a slight increase in their sex drive while on treatment with levodopa. It can be a worrying symptom, especially in the elderly, if not forewarned.

Perhaps the commonest side-effect of levodopa is a feeling of nausea with occasional vomiting. This is substantially reduced in the case of drugs containing a decarboxylase inhibitor, but may remain troublesome, particularly when treatment is first started. It is best avoided by always taking the dose after meals or at least never on an empty stomach. Nausea may result from taking an inadequate quantity of decarboxylase inhibitor at the lower levels of dosage in preparations such as Sinimet. Paradoxically, therefore, nausea and vomiting may improve when the dose is increased. So do not be put off levodopa treatment by symptoms of nausea and vomiting. Most patients – if they persevere – derive great benefit from the drug, even if they need additional treatment to suppress the nausea.

Another related effect of levodopa – caused by reducing appetite – may be some weight loss. However, this is seldom more than ten per cent of total body weight and, of course, many patients consider such an effect an advantage. A feature that is occasionally remarked upon, particularly by relatives, is that the patient develops a rather wide-eyed, startled appearance. This results from a direct action of levodopa on the eyelids and eye muscles, and it has no medical significance whatsoever.

The major side-effects of levodopa treatment are long-term, and are seldom evident at an early stage. There is an understandable tendency therefore to raise the dose of levodopa too high. Sometimes, the patient is tempted to increase the dosage on his own initiative because of the greater improvement that can be obtained in this way. However, high-dosage levodopa treatment increases the incidence of major side-effects at a later stage so it is important to keep the dose as low as possible.

The result of long-term exposure to high dosages of levodopa is that the brain changes its response mechanisms, and becomes increasingly resistant to treatment, with the development of 'swings', in which the response varies, often with remarkable suddenness, from a state characterized by severe abnormal involuntary movements to a state of severe rigidity and slowness of movement (see Appendix 1). Variation of response of this type constitutes one of the major problems of levodopa treatment in the parkinsonian patient. It can often be helped by frequent smaller doses of levodopa or by changing other aspects of treatment, but once these side-effects have developed it is rarely possible to suppress them completely.

The abnormal movements caused by these 'swings' are seldom the cause of great distress to the patient, although relatives may be only too conscious of this side-effect and embarrassed by it. The movements are typically writhing movements of the limbs or trunk, or chewing and licking movements of the mouth with grimacing of the face. If these movements are so severe as to interfere with balance or walking they obviously outweigh the benefits of the treatment and a reduction in dose becomes mandatory. Because most patients prefer to put up with abnormal movements if they can thereby be freed from the slowness of movement, it is important to understand that abnormal movements usually indicate too high a dose of levodopa, and the need for a reduction in dose if eventual loss of benefit from this drug is to be avoided.

The period of action of a single dose of levodopa is about four hours, so during the day treatment should be taken, roughly speaking, after each main meal. It follows that before the first dose in the morning symptoms are likely to be at their maximum. It is sometimes necessary therefore to take the first dose of the day after an early morning cup of tea and before attempting to dress, wash or shave. Try to time doses so that the greatest benefit is obtained at those times of day when physical activity needs to be at a maximum. There is no sense in taking levodopa at night before going to bed, and it is often unnecessary in the evening if at that time you are going to be sitting at home.

Many patients find that the period of action of levodopa reduces with the passage of time, so that eventually no benefit is noticeable for half-an-hour after taking the dose. Even then there is only notice-able benefit for about an hour before abnormal movements or slowness of movement return and another dose is required. I have patients who have to take their treatment every one or two hours through the day. It should be emphasized that nowhere in the treatment of Parkinson's disease is there greater variation than in patient's response to levodopa treat-ment after they have been taking this treatment for a few years. Each individual response needs to be assessed with great care, so that fine adjustments of dosage and timing can obtain the maximum benefit in the individual case over the long term. It will greatly help your doctor to advise you if you can tell him precisely how variations in your condition during the day relate to the timing of individual doses of levodopa.

Painful cramp (dystonic spasm) affecting especially the muscles of the calf or foot is a late side-effect of levodopa treatment. It usually is worst in the early part of the day, when it may interfere with walking and lead to considerable discomfort. Many patients, though, find that they can 'walk off' this side-effect, and it is seldom an indication for altering dosage. In some cases it is necessary to try additional treatment to relieve the dystonic spasm. The drug which is most effective for this purpose is baclofen.

Anticholinergics

Generally, anticholinergics are about half as effective as levodopa drugs. Their advantage, however, is that in early or mild cases of Parkinson's disease, their side-effects are less than those of levodopa, while their action is quite sufficient to overcome the symptoms. They are therefore very useful either early after the diagnosis, or when used in conjunction with levodopa.

A large number of proprietary anticholinergic preparations are now available; a list of these with their proprietary names can be found in Appendix 2. There is little difference in the effectiveness of these various preparations. The most widely used are benzhexol (Artane) and orphenadrine (Disipal).*

The major function of anticholinergic drugs is to relieve stiffness of the muscles. They often allow greatly improved freedom of movement and patients whose primary symptom has been difficulty in the use of one hand often report substantial benefit after starting treatment with benzhexol. Tremor may also improve with anticholinergic treatment, and benefit lasts for about four hours after each dose. But the more severe manifestations of slowness of movement and disturbance of balance seldom respond dramatically to anticholinergic drugs. Patients with the class of secondary disease known as post-encephalitic parkinsonism (see Chapter 1) will tolerate very high doses of

---

*Drug names in the text beginning with a capital letter are proprietary names. The proper chemical name of a drug is generally used in the text for preference without capitals.

anticholinergics with little or no side-effects. These drugs are therefore particularly useful in the few patients with that variety of parkinsonism.

There are two distinct groups of side-effects from anticholinergic drugs: firstly, the 'peripheral' side-effects, dryness of the mouth, blurring of near vision and slowness and hesitancy in passing water; secondly the 'central side-effects', confusion, memory impairment and hallucinations. It must be emphasized that all these side-effects are mild and the more serious ones are relatively rare. Remember that the benefits of treatment far outweigh the side-effects.

Dryness of the mouth can be unpleasant and troublesome, particularly when associated with the disturbance of taste produced by levodopa. In patients who dribble, dryness of the mouth may be a benefit, but many patients find that the thick, sticky saliva that results from anticholinergic drugs is difficult to get accustomed to. Some relief may be obtained by sipping from a glass of water or sucking acid-drop sweets.

The blurring of vision is a symptom which is most noticeable when treatment is first started. It tends to improve with time, and seldom constitutes a deterioration which demands a change of reading glasses. Any severe alteration of vision while taking anticholinergic drugs could indicate the development of glaucoma, and should be immediately reported to the doctor.

Difficulty with starting to pass water may be another side-effect of anticholinergic drugs, and may of course prevent their use altogether, especially in anybody with a history of prostate trouble. A past history of glaucoma or prostate trouble should always be reported to the general practitioner or specialist *before* treatment is prescribed.

Constipation may also be made worse by anticholinergics, but the control of constipation remains as
normal (described in Chapter 6), and it is seldom
necessary to reduce or stop anticholinergic treatment
for this reason.

The central side-effects of these drugs may cause
very serious problems, especially in the elderly, and
provide an important reason for reducing or even
withdrawing treatment. Many patients notice that their
memory for events in the recent past, or for names and
appointments, is impaired when they start anticholinergic treatment. With some minor commonsense
adjustment, however, it may be possible to overcome
the difficulty, which in any case may improve with
continuing treatment. More serious is the development
of hallucinations; this normally indicates the need to
stop anticholinergic treatment, and then hallucinations
gradually go away. Examples of hallucinations are
figures of people – either recognizable or strange and
usually threatening – or insects or animals in the room
which cannot be seen by anyone else. Occasionally
more complex delusions may occur, with the patient
convinced that they are being persecuted or influenced
by some outside force, or that their spouse or child is
misbehaving in some way.

The side-effects described above can always be
prevented by reducing the dose or adding some
additional treatment. It is therefore important to draw
your doctor's attention to any side-effects that you
notice, and ask his advice how they are best avoided.

Amantadine ('Symmetrel')

Amantadine is a drug which should be classified as dopaminergic, because it works by releasing dopamine in the brain. It can therefore be used with benefit in association with the anticholinergic drugs; in fact, it is more like the latter group in that it is a relatively mild drug whose action tends to wear off in many patients after three or four months. It is most useful therefore in the mild early case.

Amantadine has a range of action similar to levodopa, but it is much less effective. There is no increase in benefit in doses above 300mg daily, so that normally the dose should be kept below this level.

Amantadine does have the side-effect of tending to increase swelling of the feet and ankles. Patients who have a severe problem with swollen ankles should report this to their doctor. Amantadine also causes an unusual but entirely benign skin rash, which affects predominantly the thighs and forearms. The rash is called *Livedo reticularis*, and looks like a network pattern of purplish lines. It is painless but can be quite disfiguring. Some patients also suffer some degree of mental confusion and vagueness as a result of taking amantadine and again this complication means that the treatment must be stopped.

Bromocriptine, pergolide and lisuride

These are the most recently introduced forms of treatment and are chemically manufactured levodopa substitutes, which hopefully bring the same benefits without the side-effects. Importantly, however, this

45

does not mean that they represent any particular improvement over better established treatment with levodopa or anticholinergics. On the contrary, they are so new that more experience is required with these drugs before their proper role in the treatment of Parkinson's disease can be fully evaluated.

Some patients benefit from the addition of these drugs to their treatment when severe 'swings' have developed in response to levodopa. This is because the duration of action of bromocriptine and pergolide is slightly longer than levodopa. Whereas levodopa has a period of action of three or four hours, bromocriptine may last as long as six hours. If the drugs are taken together a 'smoother' response may be obtained without the violent swings mentioned earlier.

In other cases these drugs are better tolerated than levodopa with the same or greater benefits and fewer side-effects. It would, however, be unusual for these drugs to be recommended except on specialist advice from a neurologist with experience of them, because side-effects can be severe. It is not uncommon for these drugs to lead to an increase of abnormal movements, and once again confusional states may be provoked, sometimes more severe and persistent than those associated with other parkinsonian drugs.

Deprenil or selegiline

This drug has an entirely different mode of action to those so far discussed. Instead of acting itself on the nervous system, it works by blocking the breakdown of levodopa in the brain. In this way, deprenil increases the effect of levodopa and prolongs its action. Unfortunately, it often has the effect of increasing the severity and duration of side-effects of levodopa, so that it is often necessary to reduce the dose of levodopa by about a third when the drug is started, and make subsequent adjustments according to response. Some patients derive useful prolongation of the benefits of levodopa therapy, so that this drug is especially useful in patients who have to take frequent small doses of levodopa. It can sometimes lead to increased activity and alertness, so that it should normally be taken in the morning if insomnia is to be avoided.

Other drugs

Reference has already been made to the frequency and severity of depression associated with Parkinson's disease, and drugs to treat this condition are sometimes involved in the treatment. The antidepressant drugs most commonly used, a group called the tricyclics, have a mild anticholinergic action in addition to their antidepressant action. This side-effect therefore becomes beneficial in Parkinson's disease and these drugs are extremely useful in treating any depressed parkinsonian. Some tricyclic antidepressants have a sedative action, and may also be useful where insomnia is a problem.

As we have seen, tremor tends to get worse in response to nervous tension or stress. A group of drugs called the 'beta-blockers' specifically prevents the bodily manifestations of the stress reaction. These drugs may usefully reduce tremor, although the response is seldom more than about thirty per cent. The action of these drugs, however, may be particularly valuable if they are taken in preparation for a particularly stressful event – a wedding or a speech, for example. Side-effects include faint feelings, dizziness and wheezing of the chest. These drugs, like all those mentioned in this chapter, must only be taken on medical advice.

It is important, at all times, to stick carefully to the dosage and timing of any drug recommended by your doctor. Never be tempted by the idea that 'you can't have too much of a good thing' – and hence take more medication than has been advised.

Medical treatment for Parkinson's disease is remarkably effective and most patients can be relieved of all their disabling symptoms by the careful adjustment of their medication by their doctor. Finally, do not be alarmed by the side-effects described in this chapter. For the most part they are mild and improve with continuing treatment.

5

Physiotherapy and Exercise

The importance of regular exercise can scarcely be over-emphasized in Parkinson's disease. There is a very natural and understandable tendency in anyone suffering from a condition which limits mobility to reduce the amount they do. Sympathetic friends and relatives are anxious to help, and in no time the pattern of life can change from one where a relatively normal existence was possible with some effort to one where independence has been at least partly lost and far too much time is spent sitting down inactive in both body and mind. Unfortunately, once the diagnosis has been made, even the doctor may give you the impression that the treatment of the disease is a medical matter and one where you have little or no responsibility. 'Just keep taking the tablets' is a well-known phrase but in Parkinson's disease, in fact, the treatment consists of much more.

The title of this chapter may suggest some complicated, formalized system of exercises especially designed for the Parkinson's disease patient. While there are exercises which are used in this way, the word physiotherapy is being used here to describe *all* those forms of physical activity that lead to benefit for this disease.

It will be clear from the earlier description of symptoms that slowness of movement is the one which leads to the greatest disability. Indeed, in a survey for the Parkinson's Disease Society, Marie Oxtoby reported that only one patient in ten was free of handicap while on treatment. The need for something more than just 'the pills' is therefore evident, but only some seventeen per cent of all the patients she surveyed with Parkinson's disease had ever received a course of physiotherapy treatment. The availability of physiotherapy is very limited and inevitably has to be rationed, so that it is restricted to those who are likely to obtain the greatest benefit. In the case of Parkinson's disease, formal physiotherapy is most beneficial when recovering mobility that has been lost: either as the result of a period of enforced bed rest or an operation or injury for example, or as the disease has gradually led to serious immobility but where a new initiative with a combination of therapies could lead to a new activity. In either case, a course of physiotherapy lasting about three months, with sessions up to three times weekly, is fully adequate. There is no advantage in continuing physiotherapy as a way of life beyond that.

But let us start at the beginning. What about the early case? What can you do to help yourself and obtain the greatest possible benefit from the tablets? We must never forget that the tablets only work if you take advantage of their benefits. The patient with Parkinson's disease who sits in a chair and waits for his tablets to work will wait a very long time. A programme of regular daily exercise should be drawn up and followed. This has to be appropriate to the particular level of disability. At the bottom of the ladder, the patient who has only slight slowing of voluntary movement should aim to take a walk of about one mile every day. In addition, at least once a day, preferably half an hour after the first dose of the day's treatment, the neck, trunk and limb muscles should be exercised. In this way a loosening up of joints and muscles can be achieved which will tend to counteract pain and stiffness and maintain flexibility. It also has a beneficial effect on the heart and lungs; digestion is improved and constipation becomes much less troublesome.

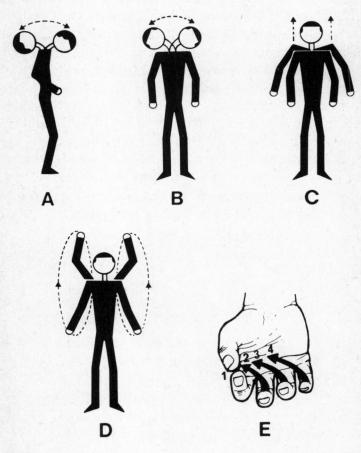

Figure 2

51

General exercises

A simple programme of exercise is as follows:-

1   Standing (See illustration on page 51)

   a. Extend and then flex your neck so that you are first looking at the ceiling and then have your chin on your chest. Repeat five times.

   b. Tilt head from side to side so that first one ear and then the other is touching the shoulder. Repeat twice on each side.

   c. Shrug both shoulders to the ears and then let them drop. Repeat five times.

   d. Raise both arms above head forwards and bring them down sideways. Repeat ten times.

   e. Practise each finger touching the top of the thumb. Repeat with each hand separately three times.

   f. Tap the hand on a table as fast as possible, each hand separately. Repeat five or ten seconds each.

Fig. 2: A, B, C, D, E.

2 Sitting on a chair without arms

   a. Tilt trunk as far as possible to one side and then the other. Repeat ten times.

   b. Lean forward, slide to the front edge of the seat and stand up. Then sit down. Don't worry if you have to cheat and have a little help with a steadying hand from a friend. Repeat five times.

Fig. 3: A, B.

3 Lying on the bed or floor

Lift one leg in the air, bending the knee, and then try to

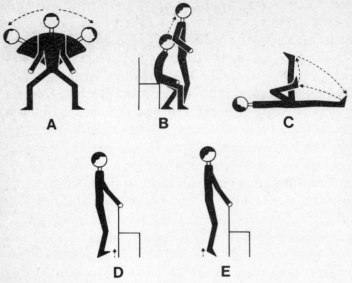

Figure 3

straighten it with the toe pointing to the ceiling. Lower to the floor and repeat with other leg. Repeat five times with each leg.

Fig. 3: C.

4 Standing and holding the back of a firm chair
Stand on tiptoe; then change so that you are standing on your heels with toes in the air. Repeat five times.

Fig. 3: D, E.

Try to do all these exercises rhythmically – it might help to do them to music. With adequate pauses for rest they can be easily accomplished within fifteen minutes. If possible they should be repeated later in the day, either after the midday dose of treatment or after the evening medication. Exercises of this type do nobody harm, and besides avoiding disruption in the home it gives encouragement and moral support if the wife or husband joins in with the patient and they do exercises together.

Sports which involve 'natural' levels of exercise and physical recreation are all of great benefit. Many of my patients continue to play golf as soon as they have made the mental adjustment to their standard of play not being what it was. One patient assured me that he got ample exercise by conducting an orchestra – as well as an enor- mous amount of artistic and social pleasure! Tennis, bowls and crocquet are all good exercise. Simple walking is excellent, and I have sometimes encouraged patients to get a dog so that the pet will encourage master or mistress to go for a walk every day.

These activities not only have a physical effect, but also get you out of the house enabling you to meet people and continue as before. It is up to relatives to give plenty of encouragement in this direction. Many patients with Parkinson's disease find it difficult or embarrassing to take the initiative to join a bowls club or look for a pet, but if a friend makes the initial enquiries and then provides the necessary encourage- ment, great good may come out of it. However – don't nag the patient to do more than he can.

Exercises for specific problems

For the patient whose mobility has been severely affected by the problems of start hesitancy, difficulties with balance and problems with turning round, these are some useful hints.

Problem 1
Start hesitancy – feet seem stuck to the floor so that you can't get going.

Solution
Don't try to walk.

Mark time by lifting each foot at least six inches off the floor, then imagine there is a brick just in front of your feet. (If you like, practise with a real brick.) *Step over it* and then . . . Keep walking, aiming to lengthen each pace by three inches beyond your natural inclination.

If you become completely stuck and can't mark time, get a friend to stand beside you. They should take you by one shoulder, and rock you gently from side to side on your feet at a rate of twice a second. This will shift your weight first on to one foot and then the other. When you feel your weight on your (say) left foot lift the right foot and you can step over the imaginary brick as before.

Problem 2
Balance disturbed – walking paces become smaller and smaller until you are leaning so far forward that you topple over and fall.

Solution
Choose a regularly patterned carpet in a corridor; or draw chalk lines eighteen inches apart along the pavement; or put down on the carpet strips of paper every eighteen inches.

Practise walking so that each pace is eighteen inches long and you have to step out to the pattern (or over the chalk mark or strips of paper).

Problem 3
Unable to turn round – knees tend to give way and feet stick.

Solution

Stop trying to turn round.

Get your balance.

Start to mark time or rock as in Problem 1, and when your feet are unstuck, turn round like a soldier stamping your feet down between each pace.

Problem 4

Balance – tendency to topple over backwards.

Solution

Carry something reasonably heavy in one or both hands; a heavy walking stick or walking frame is the obvious answer, but I have had a patient who liked to carry a heavy book and another who used a large handbag.

Note: many aluminium walking frames are much too light for people with this problem. Some of the wheeled varieties are satisfactory, or a 'Zimmer' frame can be weighted with a basket attached to the top rail. Some patients find a wheeled tea trolley best of all!

It will be clear from some of the suggestions made above that there is considerable scope for ingenuity. If you can design something that helps your problem perhaps it will help others, whom you may meet at Parkinson's Disease Society meetings.

Keeping up the exercises

Formal physiotherapy, when it can be arranged in a hospital department, is of particular benefit to patients who are lacking in confidence and need encouragement. Such patients need to be shown what they are capable of, and also need to be taught how to use walking sticks or walking frames. At the end of a course of physiotherapy it is useful if the physiotherapist makes out a list of exercises, to be done at home without supervision, which are particularly suited to the individual's needs. An occasional check-up by the physiotherapist to ensure that progress is being maintained is very beneficial – bad habits can be corrected, and the discipline of doing exercises at home is reinforced if you know that you are going to be monitored.

Every little bit of improvement that is achieved by medical treatment or physiotherapy must be used. Activities that have been abandoned must be restarted – the patient who gave up gardening or exercising the dog should try to return to these activities as soon as his physical condition allows. In this way, improvement leads to further improvement. Similarly, tasks such as writing or preparing food, or hobbies such as woodwork or painting, should be taken up again as soon as the treatment allows you to overcome the symptoms. Even helping a little with some of the cleaning or gardening is better than leaving it all to someone else.

Speech therapy

Of the physical therapies, physiotherapy is the most important, but speech therapy has a place in the management of those cases where speech difficulties are disabling. In Parkinson's disease speech may become weak and soft, and sometimes the patient cannot sustain sufficient volume to make himself heard in normal conversation. In addition there is a tendency to speak too fast, so that the words tumble out almost on top of each other, and a single word or phrase may be repeated involuntarily several times – a complaint known as palilalia. If dribbling is a problem, it too clearly complicates speech difficulty.

There is much that can be done to improve speech abnormalities. The first stage is for the patient to be fully and critically aware of what the problem is. If you can use a tape recorder and listen to yourself this is a good start. Practise increasing the volume by reading out loud and concentrating on each word so that the voice is not allowed to fade away, and practise the rhythm of speech by consciously slowing down and introducing short pauses between words. It is also a good idea to try singing in accompaniment to a disc or tape. Try to take deep breaths while speaking. Some patients find it helpful to watch themselves in a mirror while doing these exercises.

Where speech difficulties are especially severe, referral to a professional speech therapist should be requested. Like physiotherapy, speech therapy is usually best given as an introductory course with occasional subsequent reassessment for further corrective therapy.

There are now some electronic gadgets available which may help patients with severe speech difficulty. The simplest is a speech amplifier – a loudspeaker – which means you can turn up the volume artificially. Some patients with palilalia (stammering or very rapid speech) have been helped by apparatus which delivers a momentarily delayed auditory feedback. In patients who, through severe Parkinson's disease, have lost the power of speech altogether, small portable typewriters may enable them to communicate by typing out a message on a paper strip. These 'communicators' are costly if bought privately but can usually be obtained through the NHS on a consultant's recommendation.

Home adjustments and aids and appliances

Consider realistically what changes in your home environment would make life easier. I would suggest that you begin by asking what would you be better to do without before considering what additional aids might help. For instance, there is no sense in continuing to live with lots of small mats and rugs if you shuffle and tend to catch your feet on them.

Let us start with clothing. Buttons may be difficult and best replaced with velcro or zips. Shoelaces are awkward – elastic sided slip-on shoes are better. Leather soles are less likely to catch on the ground and cause stumbling than crepe rubber, and it is often helpful anyway when walking to be able to hear the leather sole on the floor. Patients who tend to topple backwards may be helped by higher heels or a heel rise inside the shoe. A heel of 1–1½ inches is about right, and the heel should be broad enough to give support and balance. Those tending to fall forwards should select shoes with little or no heel.

Sticks and walking frames have already been discussed, but around the house handles attached to door frames or suitably placed near bath and toilet are better to steady yourself and retain independence. In general, use chairs that are high and upright because most parkinsonians find low reclining easy chairs impossible to get out of. Gadgets are available for raising the height of chairs with wooden legs. Some patients find it helpful to tilt their chair forwards by raising the back legs two or three inches. Spring-loaded seats are useful so long as the patient can step forward, as they are lifted, by the special seat. In some cases a tendency to slide down in the chair can be prevented by sitting on a rubber ring. Lavatory seats tend to be much too low and seats which raise the level of the lavatory are available and often a great help.

One of the commonest complaints is the inability to turn over in bed. This may be helped by using a duvet instead of blankets, and slippery nylon sheets instead of cotton ones. Some patients like to have an upright chair with its back to the bedside which they can grasp to pull themselves over. Others find a loop of rope lying on the top of the bed and tied to the legs at the foot of the bed enables them to sit up and move about in bed. Like the chair, a high bed is easier to get out of than a low one, and a firm mattress easier to turn on than a soft one.

At meal times it is easier to use cutlery with relatively thick handles. Non-slip mats under the plate often help. If tremor results in liquids being spilt a straw or drinking mug with a spout is often useful.

When writing, and as with cutlery, a pen that is thick enough to grasp easily may help. But if writing is very difficult, don't give up correspondence; it is much better to continue writing to friends and dealing with essential correspondence by using a typewriter.

The appliances mentioned in this section are available from your local authority Social Services department, on loan from the Red Cross, or can be bought at some of the useful addresses at the end of this book. But the suggestions made here are perhaps just a start. Each individual is faced with individual problems, and ingenuity as to how best to solve them will achieve much more than recommendations made by someone with no knowledge of your individual case.

6

Diet and Daily Living

Special diets, the science of dietetics and dietary supplements with vitamins and the like have long enjoyed publicity in the media. It is natural, therefore, to ask whether Parkinson's disease may be caused by some dietary deficiency or excess, or whether treatment may be improved by some dietary restriction or supplement. In general, the answer must be that diet has no known effect on the cause of Parkinson's disease and dietary considerations play a relatively small part in the management of this condition. Nevertheless, it is worth looking at these matters in a little more detail.

It is true that in South America and elsewhere a form of parkinsonism exists which is caused by excessive absorption of manganese (in miners working with manganese salts) but this is a very rare phenomenon and careful investigation has failed to implicate manganese – or any other constituent of food – in the cause of Parkinson's disease in the developed western countries. Moreover, the incidence of the disease is relatively constant in countries with widely differing dietary habits, and there is nothing to suggest that modern processed food has any part in causing the disease. Low animal-fat diets have recently been recommended especially for those with heart or arterial diseases, but there is nothing to suggest that such diets protect the individual from Parkinson's disease.

So are there then any special pieces of dietary advice that should be given to someone suffering from Parkinson's disease? The answer is that diet may have some effect on response to treatment; and constipation and obesity are two common problems in Parkinson's disease where diet is obviously relevant.

The normal action of levodopa may be affected by high protein levels in the diet. A meal containing large quantities of meat, fish or cheese, for example, may reduce the absorption of levodopa (even in combination with decarboxylase inhibitor) and thereby reduce the benefit of treatment. This effect is purely temporary, so that you may discover from your own observations that you are more stiff and slowed up if you eat a large meal of steak or hamburger. However, it is important not to go to the opposite extreme and avoid protein. The ideal is simply a consistent and regular diet containing a normal amount of meat or fish, so that the dose of levodopa can be adjusted to match the diet and thereby avoid too severe a day-to-day variation in response. It is probably similarly preferable to make the midday meal lighter than the evening meal, so that the main meal of the day can include more protein without the ensuing effects seriously interfering with the day's activity.

Vitamin B6 (pyridoxine), when taken as a vitamin supplement in large amounts, will interfere with levodopa if it is being taken without decarboxylase inhibitor. With drugs such as Madopar or Sinemet, no such effect occurs, but nevertheless it is probably preferable not to take vitamin B6 in tablet form. The quantities of B6 in foods such at Marmite, Bovril, wheat-germ, liver and tomatoes will not have any harmful effects.

Diet is important, however, as far as it affects general physical condition. Parkinson's disease often develops at a time of life when people have a weight problem, and being overweight certainly makes the symptoms and management of Parkinson's disease more difficult. It is obvious that obesity slows you up, makes you more breathless and leads to greater fatigue after only moderate exercise. It is also important, but less widely known, that obesity greatly increases the wear and tear on the hip and knee joints, and the painful osteoarthritis that results may seriously interfere with mobility already limited by Parkinson's disease. There is therefore much to be said for aiming to get into good physical shape as part of the programme of treatment, and the only safe and satisfactory way to lose weight is by a reducing diet. Fortunately, the treatment given for Parkinson's disease often reduces appetite and makes it much easier to stick to a reducing diet. The increased physical activity that results from successful treatment will also help to reduce weight. Maintenance of a normal body weight in those who tend to put on weight is a matter of continuous vigilance so, if you have a weight problem, weigh yourself regularly and be strict with your diet before excessive weight gain has occurred. It is always easier to avoid putting on weight in the first place than to lose it afterwards.

Just occasionally, and especially in the elderly, weight loss becomes a problem. This may result from some associated medical condition so you should always consult your doctor in this situation. But if some stimulation of appetite is required a drug useful for this purpose and which has anti-parkinsonian properties is Periactin (cyproheptadine). Dietary supplements with milk drinks containing, for example, 'Build-up' or 'Complan' may also be useful.

Constipation

Constipation is a symptom of Parkinson's disease and, as has already been mentioned (see pages 27 and 44), it tends to be made worse by anticholinergic treatment. However, it is important not to overestimate the problem – constipation is a nuisance but seldom leads to serious complications. It should ideally be managed by paying attention to relatively simple adjustments in diet and fluid intake, and increasing exercise and physical activity. So the aim should be to take a 'high fibre' diet containing: plenty of fruit, especially plums, prunes and figs; nuts and raisins; green and root vegetables; wholemeal bread and bran-containing cereals. Every meal should contain at least some of these items. Very often no additional laxative treatment is required, provided fluid intake is adequate and regular daily exercise maintained. I always advise patients to drink at least one glass of water with each main meal.

Where such measures prove inadequate, laxatives must be used, but we should first of all be clear that constipation cannot precisely be defined. For some a bowel motion twice weekly is normal whereas others require a daily motion. Laxatives should rarely be used if the bowels move at least three times a week.

There are three types of laxative treatment for constipation in Parkinson's disease. The first and most important are the bulk purgatives similar in their action to the high-fibre foods described above, which work by introducing into the diet large amounts of fibre or roughage. Thus bran may be purchased and added to food or taken as tablets (Fybranta). Fybogel, Isogel, Regulan or Normacol are alternative bulk purgatives commercially prepared as granules or powder to be taken in water two or three times daily. Closely related to the bulk purgatives are the osmotic laxatives, such as Milk of Magnesia or liver salts which can be obtained without a prescription. The danger of these osmotic laxatives is that they may lead to a watery diarrhoea, and often cause incontinence.

The second group, known as the irritant laxatives, are the wide range of drugs which are obtainable without prescription. Cascara, Dulcolax, senna and Dorbanex are examples from this group, as are neostigmine or pyridostigmine, which are prescribed by the doctor and may be used in the treatment of constipation in Parkinson's disease. A small regular dose taken last thing at night is probably the ideal routine, with the aim of a motion after breakfast the next day.

The third group of laxatives – the lubricant laxatives – are less useful in most patients. Liquid paraffin should probably be avoided because it may interfere with the absorption in the bowel of other drugs being given for Parkinson's disease. However, there is one of this group, dioctyl sodium, which may be a useful laxative in some patients.

One final word about constipation: if severe and intractable, it may lead to two complications. First, there may be restlessness and confusion at night, especially in the elderly. Secondly, it may result in hesitancy and even retention of the bladder or, at the other extreme, incontinence of urine, especially at night. Attention to constipation should therefore be an early consideration where these problems develop.

Drinking and smoking during treatment

Patients often ask whether they are allowed to smoke and drink alcohol, or whether it will accelerate their disease or interfere with treatment. These activities, in moderation, are perfectly safe. Alcohol does not react with the drugs prescribed for Parkinson's disease – indeed, many people find that a small nightcap helps them sleep better.

Sleep

After constipation, difficulties with sleep are among the more common worries, but again insomnia seldom leads to any complication or real disability. Nevertheless, to be unable to turn over or get comfortable is an unpleasant experience. It is generally advisable not to take deprenil in the afternoon or levodopa within three hours of going to bed, because these drugs may cause difficulties in getting to sleep. A warm drink, and perhaps something stronger, as mentioned above, is often the ideal solution, but sedative drugs may be necessary. In this case drugs such as glutethimide (commercially available as Doriden), chloral hydrate (as a draught or tablet called Weldorm) or chlormethiazole (Heminevrin) are usually more suitable than barbiturates or drugs such as diazepam, which may make the slowness of movement of Parkinson's disease worse. With any sedative drug particular care must be taken to avoid doses which lead to confusion or hallucinations at night.

Sexual activity

There is no need to feel embarrassed to ask your doctor questions about sexual activity and the effects, if any, it may have on your disability. Certainly, he or she will feel no embarrassment and may, indeed, be able to give you much reassurance. In many people no problems arise, as the condition often occurs at an age when there is, in any case, a decline of interest in sexual relationships. But this is sometimes not the case and, furthermore, treatment with drugs containing levodopa may cause a distressing stimulation of libido, or sexual desire. This type of reaction to the treatment should be discussed with your doctor, because it may indicate the need for additional drugs or a reduction in dose of levodopa.

More commonly, and especially in the younger patient, a normal sex-life continues in spite of the development of Parkinson's disease. Most patients find that there is a very marked variability in their desire for sexual intercourse, which is after all not so unusual. The physical symptoms of Parkinson's disease may limit sexual activity, however, and so it is common for the person with Parkinson's disease to have intercourse in a recumbent posture underneath their partner. But the physical activity associated with sexual intercourse is not harmful.

Finally, it is unusual for the drugs used in treatment to affect sexual performance, but if you are male and any degree of impotence develops, consult your doctor as changes in your treatment might relieve this problem.

Personal hygiene

Parkinson's disease, as we have discovered, tends to cause a slight greasiness of the skin called seborrhoea. This is improved by treatment with levodopa, but nevertheless it is important to take particular care over personal hygiene. The forehead in particular may become rather shiny with irritation and scaling so daily washing with soap and regular shampooing of the hair is advisable. A sulphur and salicylic acid cream from your doctor may be useful in the treatment of seborrhoea and a selenium sulphide shampoo may be useful for excessive dandruff.

Regular bathing may pose problems where it is difficult to manoeuvre into or out of an ordinary bath. Appropriately placed grab handles on the wall or attached to the taps of the bath may help. Alternatively a small stool in the bath, or a board across the top can be used to sit on, thereby avoiding the need to sink right down into the bath. A non-slip mat in the bath may further reduce the risk of accidents. Where mobility is severely affected a seat in a shower may be the best answer, but this method of washing is necessarily laborious, and takes as much time as a bed bath, a more thorough method of washing an immobile patient, where separate washing of each individual part is done from a bowl on the bed.

The anticholinergic drugs used to treat Parkinson's disease cause dryness of the mouth, and the reduced flow of saliva tends to lead to crusting and plaque formation on the teeth. Brushing of teeth and gum margins twice daily is an important part of routine hygiene, and regular dental treatment should be sought from the dentist at least once a year.

Interests and hobbies

The key to overcoming the effects of Parkinson's disease is to remain mentally and physically active. The problem in some ways is similar to the problems posed by retirement. There is a great temptation to proscrastinate – to put off doing things until tomorrow or the day after – or to leave them for someone else. This mental attitude must be consciously and vigorously resisted.

Similarly, all physical activity requires much greater effort, and again there is a tendency to seek the comfort and relaxation of the armchair and to avoid getting out to do the shopping or to enjoy a walk in the park or countryside. At home, preparation of meals, cleaning or home decorating may be left increasingly to others – unless the temptation is resisted. Do not resent encouragement or even nagging from your family to help with these tasks. It is much too easy to feel that this year you cannot cope with the garden when, with a lot of effort, not only can you do the work in the garden, but also you can benefit from the exercise and stimulus involved. Medical treatment in Parkinson's disease works only if it is made to work – by the patient using the benefits from the treatment to lead an active life. Your armchair is your enemy and the less time you spend in it the better.

It would be impossible to list all the hobbies and interests suitable for someone with Parkinson's disease. Golf, bowls, croquet, walking and swimming are just some of the sports that are often suitable and enjoyable. A friend, a pub or a library to visit may establish a useful routine. Gardening, home decorating and carpentry, as well as some of the routine food preparation and home cleaning (for both sexes), maintains activity, interest and involvement. Discourage your family from taking over these routine tasks – they may feel guilty allowing you to pull your weight, but within what you can do and help with, all physical activity is a help.

Mental activity is just as important as physical activity. The tremor or the abnormal movements which may complicate treatment lead to embarrassment, and many people avoid social contact as a result. This is a tragedy, because social isolation leads to an increasingly introspective and apathetic attitude, whereas meeting friends is stimulating and keeps you mentally active. To entertain friends or family regularly provides the necessary stimulus and break with routine.

The Parkinson's Disease Society has branches in most parts of the country and deserves support from all patients with Parkinson's disease. The branches of the Society organize meetings in the winter and outings in the summer, all an excellent opportunity to get out and meet people with similar problems. There is the chance to discover ways of solving problems you may have come up against or merely to exchange ideas, and these meetings often make you realize that you are not the only one with a problem. When you support the Parkinson's Disease Society you also know that you are supporting an organization devoted to helping people like you with Parkinson's disease, and furthering research into discovering new ways of improving the treatment of people with this condition.

7

Work and Driving

While many patients develop their first symptoms of Parkinson's disease after they have retired from work, some develop symptoms during their forties or fifties or even earlier, and questions naturally arise about fitness to continue work. The general principle must always be – try to continue work if at all possible, and try not to plan too far ahead.

Keeping up a job has a number of advantages. First and foremost, it imposes a discipline which maintains mental and physical activity. To have to get up at a set time in the morning is beneficial. To have to plan the routine in such a way as to be able to fit everything in before setting out to work – washing, dressing, breakfast and travel – will also encourage a positive attitude towards coping with the symptoms of the disease. There may be those at home and at work who take a gloomy view – they will look too far ahead and discourage you. They expect the present problems to get worse quickly, but this may very well not be so. Cross bridges only when you come to them, and don't give up a job because of what you may eventually suffer – it might never happen.

The range of specific and particular problems encountered in the work environment is obviously too wide to consider in detail here. But it is important to identify one common problem from the outset – embarrassment. The tremor of Parkinson's disease is conspicuous, and tends to attract attention under the very circumstances that are most distressing – while

71

talking in public, or sitting in a meeting. Tremor may be mistakenly identified in the minds of some people with senile decay, and it is the anticipation of this attitude that makes the parkinsonian especially anxious to conceal his tremor. But don't make the control of tremor a condition of your continuing in work, because it is rare for complete suppression of tremor to be achieved by treatment.

It is better to bring the problem out into the open. Refer to it in normal conversation, admit that you are being treated for Parkinson's disease and emphasize how little disability the tremor causes. Tell the truth – most patients find it is not severely disabling, only conspicuous and embarrassing. Once people know that you have come to terms with your tremor, they will follow suit and come to ignore it, instead of sympathizing in a patronizing and ultimately derogatory way.

You must, of course, be realistic about your symptoms and accept adjustment. If there are some aspects of your work which you find difficult through slowness of movement or softness of speech, discuss the matter with the head of your department. People are usually anxious to cooperate in reducing the stress and strain of a full working day, when this is necessary through disability. But above all stand up for yourself. I have had patients deprived of their work in an office, sorting newspapers or working as a gardener, when they were fully capable of doing everything that was required of them.

The commonest problem at work is general mobility. It may take much longer to walk to work from the bus stop or car park, and to pop into another office along the corridor may take time where previously it had been done in seconds without thinking. Stairs and steps are often difficult to negotiate, especially in a crowd of people, and it often helps to display a robust walking stick which immediately identifies your disability so that people are less likely to push or bump into you.

The person with Parkinson's disease is inevitably dependent on the understanding and help of colleagues at work, but most patients, whatever there disability, don't want the attentions of a conspicuously sympathetic 'do-gooder'. So do explain to your friends at work when their assistance can be useful. If they could carry something for you, give a helping hand down steps or into a car, change the typewriter ribbon or ballpoint refill, tell them so. An understanding, helpful attitude on both sides can make it possible to overcome problems which might otherwise prevent your continuing in work, and also builds up relationships which may be the most valuable outcome of all.

Writing is often a problem. In Parkinson's disease the sufferer tends to get slower in writing and the script tends to get untidy and progressively smaller. There may also be difficulty in placing writing on the page. In the early stages a large-barrelled pen may help, but as a rule a typewriter is the best solution even though this means that the exercise of writing is removed.

Some patients also develop a speech difficulty, and this will cause particular problems at work when the voice becomes so soft that the telephone cannot be used. This softness of speech is called dysphonia, and is often accompanied by a mumbling repetition of certain syllables reminiscent of stammering. The latter problem can sometimes be helped with speech therapy, but dysphonia usually requires a voice amplifier or loudspeaker. These can be successfully used in conjunction with the telephone – indeed many patients find voice

73

amplifiers embarrassing to use in face to face conversation but lose their inhibitions on the telephone.

Perhaps the commonest problem of all is simple fatigue. A day's work which, in the past, would not have seemed exceptional leaves the parkinsonian exhausted and completely without the will to do anything constructive when he or she returns home in the evening. This fatigue must be accepted as part of the disease, and taken into account when deciding what changes to make in the working routine. In most cases, shift work has to be avoided and the hours of work reduced.

If the point is reached where you are no longer able to continue work, premature retirement can be sought on medical grounds. In this way, your pension rights are protected and sickness benefit remains payable until you are of pensionable age. It will be necessary to get a letter from your doctor for the personnel department at work, stating that, in your doctor's opinion, continuing at work will be undesirable for medical reasons, and that retirement on medical grounds is recommended.

It may be helpful and therapeutic to maintain an active interest in some aspect of your work after retirement, or, if this is not possible, to take up voluntary work (possibly with your local branch of the Parkinson's Disease Society) to keep your mind active and utilize your talents.

Driving

The ability to continue to work is often dependent on using a car to get there, or even to carry out the job. Travel by bus or train poses particular problems for the parkinsonian, as high steps have to be negotiated, and a bus is likely to move and throw you off balance before you are sitting down.

The regulations in the United Kingdom governing medical fitness to drive are precise and there are similar regulations in most countries. Any condition which may cause a relevant disability and which is expected to last more than three months must be reported to the Driver and Vehicle Licensing Centre. A decision will then be made as to how often the medical review of fitness to drive should be undertaken. The responsibility for reporting disability rests with the patient, and the responsibility for deciding if a patient is medically fit rests with the family doctor, advised by the neurologist.

The doctor's decision is seldom an easy one. The patient is always very aware that continuing to drive enables him to retain mobility, to avoid imposing on family and friends for transport, and even in many cases to continue at work or at least maintain many outside interests. But the doctor has to put aside all personal considerations in favour of his primary duty to prevent danger to the public from a patient driving when medically unfit. Patients often plead that they will only drive short distances, or very slowly; or they may point out that the car is their only means of doing the shopping. But if the doctor believes that his patient is unfit he must set such considerations aside and say so, because the stress of driving on someone medically unfit is harmful, and tends to make their parkinsonian symptoms worse; and of course the effects – physical and psychological – of a crash can be devastating. We know that the symptoms of Parkinson's disease are worse following an illness such as flu or a bad cold, or after a surgical operation. It may take many weeks for the normal level of benefit achieved by treatment to be regained. Similarly, injury from a road traffic accident will set a patient back in a way that may be difficult or impossible to regain.

The decision over fitness to drive is one that should be discussed fully and frankly with your doctor. If you are confident of your safety and competence, and if someone who knows your driving skills well can confirm that the disease has not affected your driving, then this information should be given to your doctor because he will certainly take these points into careful consideration. You should always notify your motor insurance company of the diagnosis and of the doctor's decision.

If the disease progresses, and you have to give up driving later on, this is another situation where a positive approach is needed. You must decide how to reorganize your travel arrangements, and it is surprising how many taxi fares you can get out of what it costs to license and run a car.

8

The Elderly Parkinsonian

Parkinson's disease is usually a condition of middle and late life. In the last chapter we were mainly considering the problems faced by the middle-aged patient at work. Now we will look at some of the problems which face the elderly parkinsonian.

The usual problems of old age often coincide with the more intractable manifestations of Parkinson's disease. The elderly parkinsonian may have had the disease for many years, and therefore be suffering the complications of prolonged treatment, and he almost always will have the conditions associated with old age, such as arthritis, failing vision, prostate troubles and perhaps shortness of breath from chest or heart conditions. Failure of memory and mental confusion, falling and problems of walking are all more likely in any elderly person than in the young parkinsonian. On the other hand, it is an interesting and unexplained fact that cancer is significantly less common in people with Parkinson's disease than the general population of the same age.

With these complaints there inevitably comes a variety of treatments. The drugs administered for other conditions may interact with those used for the treatment of Parkinson's disease, so that it is important, especially if you come under the care of a new doctor (for example, if you are admitted to hospital for some other illness) to have a list of the drugs you are taking. The older patient is more likely to be taking a number of pills for various conditions, and when the

Parkinson's disease is first treated it is usually a good time to review these and reduce the number of different drugs to a minimum.

Arthritis

Arthritis is a word used to describe two very different conditions – rheumatoid arthritis and osteoarthritis. Rheumatoid arthritis is relatively uncommon, but may occur in association with Parkinson's disease. Osteo-arthritis, however, is so common as to afflict almost everybody over the age of sixty to some extent; it is the cause of painful stiffness of the neck or shoulder, and may cause backache. Pain in the hips and knees is also common, especially in anyone who is overweight. Osteoarthritis is actually nothing more than wear and tear, but when its painful stiffness and limitation of movement is added to the rigidity and slowness of Parkinson's disease, the combination may be very disabling. Arthritis, as distinct from Parkinson's disease, is a painful limitation of movement at a joint, which is relieved by resting the joint. As we have already seen, Parkinson's disease may cause similar pain, so that it may be difficult for the patient to judge which pain is due to which complaint. In this situation do seek expert medical advice, because it is only by carefully explaining your symptoms to your doctor and by undergoing examination (possibly with X-rays) that the matter can be properly sorted out and appropriate treatment given. It is no good taking large quantities of painkillers for inadequately treated Parkinson's disease, any more than it is to take excessive parkinsonian treatment for arthritis.

Any of the common painkillers are useful in treating

the pain of arthritis, and they do not interact with Parkinson's disease drugs. Aspirin, paracetamol, Distalgesic and drugs such as indomethacin (which has to be given under medical supervision) are all suitable. supervision) are all suitable.

Urinary problems

Urinary symptoms are particularly common in the elderly male, because enlargement of the prostate gland near the bladder is increasingly frequent around the age of sixty. This condition causes frequency – so that the patient has to pass water every one or two hours and rise at night two or even more times, and there is difficulty in starting, with a 'poor stream'.

The anticholinergic drugs used for Parkinson's disease tend to act on the muscles of the bladder and make all these difficulties worse. Furthermore, they exacerbate constipation, which of itself will make prostatic symptoms worse. Finally, in this sequence of upsets, a full or irritable bladder disturbs sleep and may lead to nightmares or confusion at night.

While the patient with prostate trouble should therefore avoid anticholinergic drugs, it is often wise to undergo appropriate surgical treatment of the prostate gland when the symptoms are still relatively mild. Prostate operations nowadays do not involve any abdominal incisions, and are much less stressful than they were fifteen or twenty years ago.

In some elderly patients a catheter, a flexible tube inserted into the urinary tract, can be the simplest and most effective answer to the problem. A catheter may also be necessary if incontinence has developed either as a complication following a prostate operation or simply because of illness and old age. While modern plastic catheters are less uncomfortable than the old rubber ones, they nevertheless have complications, especially bladder infections, and need careful medical and nursing supervision.

In the female, urinary problems most commonly relate to bladder infection. The development of incontinence in the elderly female parkinsonian may indicate a bladder infection, and again this complication may cause restlessness and confusion at night. The difficulties are especially great if the patient cannot get out of bed to reach a toilet. Symptoms of bladder infection (or cystitis) are burning pain on passing water, frequency, abdominal discomfort and worsening of the parkinsonian symptoms. The condition can usually be readily treated with appropriate antibiotics under medical supervision.

Confusion and memory failure

These are some of the most distressing and worrying problems for the elderly parkinsonian. In the old days Parkinson's disease substantially reduced life expectancy, and so these complications were much less common, but now that many patients with Parkinson's disease can expect a normal or near-normal life expectancy, confusional states, memory failure and dementia are much more frequent.

At present, relatively little can be done medically to help this problem where it is due to ageing of the brain. But a very careful search must always be made for a different cause; all the drugs used in treatment of Parkinson's disease may cause a confusional state, so the first consideration must always be to exclude the possibility that the confusion is due to one or other drug. Anticholinergics can be troublesome in this respect, and should only be used with great caution in the elderly.

The commonly used sedatives are often to blame. Sleeping pills therefore have to be chosen with very great care for the elderly patient with Parkinson's disease, and if confusion at night is associated with insomnia, medical advice should always be taken about suitable sleeping tablets. A sensible routine could avoid the need for sedatives altogether. There is an inevitable tendency for the elderly to doze in a chair during the day and then have difficulty sleeping at night. This tendency can be avoided if the daytime routine keeps mind and body active. Natural sleep resulting from the tiredness that comes at the end of an active day is far preferable to sleep induced by drugs. A warm drink and a nightcap of something alcoholic are often the most effective preludes to settling down for the night.

Most elderly people complain of failure of memory. They can usually remember events of long ago in remarkable detail, but find difficulty in recalling the recent past. This is a normal effect of ageing. In Parkinson's disease, however, another disturbance of memory may be noticed, called 'thought block'. In the middle of a conversation you suddenly find you are unable to remember what you were talking about; you lose the thread and have to pause for several seconds – perhaps being prompted by a person you were speaking to – before being able to carry on. This common symptom should not cause alarm, because it does not indicate the start of any mental decline. Neither is it usually a side-effect of any of the drugs, although occasional patients have noticed a little improvement if they stop anticholinergic drugs. Don't allow this symptom to prevent you joining in the conversation:

rather, teach your family and friends that, from time to time, they will have to prompt your memory.

A general impairment of memory and intellect known as Alzheimer's disease is common in the elderly, and occurs more frequently in patients with Parkinson's disease than in other people of the same age. So far, we have not been able to develop any form of drug treatment for this condition but there is good reason to hope that such treatment will become available in the future. At present, problems of severe failure of memory and intellect have to be managed by appropriate help and adjustment of the patient's environment. Where Alzheimer's disease and Parkinson's disease co-exist, the drugs used for the treatment of Parkinson's disease may make the mental state worse, and therefore have to be withdrawn.

It is always necessary to give higher priority to the care of the patient's overall mental state, even when the stopping of a drug leads to some loss of mobility and physical activity. In this situation the elderly and severely disabled patient will need much help. He will continue to need the encouragement to do what he can, but more important than ever is the reassurance of knowing there will always be those around him who will help and relieve suffering. At this stage the importance of nursing help and medical advice and supervision is paramount – not only to the patient but to his family. If long-term care in nursing home accommodation can be avoided, the happiness of the patient is generally much better served. But where the physical effects of untreated Parkinson's disease have produced an inability to walk, or have led to an injury such as a broken hip, nursing in bed may become essential and care in a hospital or nursing home inevitable.

9

Hope for the Future

Improvements in the treatment of Parkinson's disease over the last thirty years have been greater than for almost any other disease known to medicine. It was only that long ago that the medical textbooks described it as one of the diseases 'least amenable to therapeutic agents'. Now it is held up to medical students as a prime example of a disease where the discovery of the underlying abnormality has led to the introduction of effective treatment. Happily, we can expect even further advances if and when some of the current research yields results.

New drugs

For all the marvellous improvements made possible by levodopa, the time should come when it is replaced by even better treatments. Perhaps its major problem is its tendency to induce unpleasant side-effects, as previously detailed. These are now not accepted as an inevitable part of the treatment of Parkinson's disease, and chemists are researching into the possibility of manufacturing synthetic chemicals which have the beneficial effects of levodopa without the side-effects. Drugs like bromocriptine, pergolide and lisuride, already discussed in Chapter 4, are the first fruits of this work.

The other drawback of levodopa is that it remains effective for only about four hours, and the research to replace it is trying to find drugs that have longer-lasting benefits. In this way one or two doses a day of a new drug may give freedom from symptoms throughout twenty-four hours and avoid the 'swings' from immobility to excessive abnormal movement.

Deprenil, also described in Chapter 4, is a drug whose action depends upon a different principle – that of slowing down the breakdown of levodopa. It also prolongs the action of levodopa, and therefore helps to achieve a smoother response. Other drugs acting in the same way may be developed, or the same principle may be applied to the breakdown of synthetic drugs used for Parkinson's disease.

The problem of side-effects of levodopa developing after a patient has been on treatment for some time is probably the most serious that doctor and patient have to cope with at the moment. Much research is devoted to this problem.

What causes Parkinson's disease?

The most fundamental and, therefore, important question is the cause of Parkinson's disease. If we could find out what it is that starts the dopamine deficiency that sets the disease off in the first place, there is every likelihood that we could both prevent its development and arrest its progression.

Parkinson's disease used to be thought of as analogous to ageing, but this is no longer acceptable and it is now generally agreed that the disease has a cause or multiple causes. We now believe that the nerve cells in the brain which stop working, and thereby give rise to the symptoms of Parkinson's disease, are destroyed by some specific agent or chemical. It has been suggested that one possible treatment would be to transplant healthy brain tissue to replace that damaged by the disease, but such a form of treatment is still a long way off.

If we could discover the cause of Parkinson's disease, then it would become more essential than ever to diagnose the disease very early – before any damage had been done. One of the aims of research, therefore, is to find ways of detecting the earliest chemical changes in the brain that indicate the start of the condition. We have a large accumulation of knowledge about what does *not* cause Parkinson's disease, as we discussed in Chapter 1, including the most surprising fact that it is less common in smokers than in non-smokers – the opposite of so many diseases. As a result, the question has repeatedly been raised whether this apparent protection from the disease by a history of cigarette smoking contains the clue to the cause, but so far no plausible theory that explains this unusual relationship to smoking has been forthcoming.

There are two main theories about what causes Parkinson's disease. The first suggests that the disease is due to invasion of the nervous system by a virus, possibly many years or even decades before any sign of the disease develops. Damage to nerve cells proceeds extremely slowly and surviving cells compensate, until a critical point is reached where compensation can no longer prevent the emergence of the first symptoms of the disease.

In the second theory, a nerve poison or toxin is suggested as the agent which causes the nerve cell damage. The gradual accumulation of a metal or organic chemical in the brain slowly affects the working of the cells in the regions of the brain we know to be damaged in Parkinson's disease.

Considerable research has been directed to trying to

find either a virus particle or a toxic substance or chemical which might cause the disease in this way. But so far no agent of this kind has been discovered. Surveys of cases of Parkinson's disease have failed to show any common factor between them which might suggest similar exposure to a virus or other agent. Such research continues and it is likely that eventually a cause will be found; after all, it has been possible to demonstrate the cause of so many other less common diseases of the nervous system.

The progress in Parkinson's disease research has been so impressive that it is difficult not to expect that the remaining problems of the disease will be solved before too long. Already the disease is no longer the terrifying prospect it once was – we can now relieve most of the symptoms of Parkinson's disease in the majority of patients. With careful and continuing treatment most patients can lead active and independent lives, often without the nature of their disability being recognisable except to their family or close friends. Parkinson's disease was the first disease of the nervous system to be shown to be treatable by the replacement of a depleted chemical in the brain. With the continuation of worldwide active research we must hope that the basic cause – and hence cure – of the disease will not escape us much longer.

Appendix 1

Parkinson's Disease – A Personal Account

I am a married man in my early fifties and I have had Parkinson's disease for eighteen years. I was playing darts when I first noticed that something was wrong – my hand was trembling slightly, and the fingers gripped the dart a fraction too long so that it struck the board lower than the point aimed at. Mildly annoyed, I decided that I ought to cut down a bit on the beer. That was in 1965. The next thing to deteriorate was my handwriting. I used to have a neat, italic hand, and I also enjoyed drawing in pen and ink. My last published drawings were done in 1965. Writing became increasingly difficult, with the hand slowing down after the first few words as muscular rigidity and tremor produced the typical tiny writing.

I tried for a long time to ignore the problem, but eventually in late 1967 I went to see my GP, who referred me to an eminent neurologist. After a thorough examination the neurologist came straight to the point: I was in the early stages of a form of Parkinson's disease (he used the term 'focal parkinsonism') affecting my left arm and leg, and marked by muscle pain due to rigidity with very little tremor. He told me that it was incurable and progressive. There were drugs which could alleviate the symptoms in some cases, and brain surgery was also possible. The average life expectancy was between eight and fifteen years, but as I was considerably younger (thirty-six) than the majority of parkinsonians my prospects were probably better than that. These remarks were made, of course, before levodopa treatment had been introduced and at a time when the prospects for anyone with the disease were much worse than they are now. I was told then that I could carry on working for the time being and living a normal life, but I must expect to tire increasingly easily. In fact I continued in full-time work for another sixteen years!

My immediate reaction after this consultation was one of gratitude for the specialist's candour, and relief at his diagnosis: I knew next to nothing about parkinsonism, and had expected worse (perhaps a brain tumour). The greater difficulty was in breaking the news to my wife and to my parents.

The neurologist advised a course of treatment with Artane, which began in December 1967. I made the mistake (entirely my own fault) of starting this treatment on a day when I had to drive 150 miles to give an evening lecture. The consequences were embarrassing and nearly disastrous: double vision and hallucinations during the drive, slurred and incoherent speech in the lecture. It was my first experience of the effect of anti-parkinsonian drugs on the brain. After a few weeks it became clear that in my case the benefits to be gained from Artane were more than outweighed by the bad side-effects, and the treatment was discontinued. There followed nearly four years without treatment, during which my activities were very gradually limited by increasing rigidity and fatigue.

In the autumn of 1971 treatment with Brocadopa (levodopa) was started. The beneficial effects were rapid and dramatic, seeming to justify for once the 'miracle drug' label which the press inevitably used. For the first time in years I felt vigorous, creative and relaxed. My writing became much more legible and its speed increased more than fourfold. By Christmas I could draw again with relative facility. In order to maintain the improvement, however, it proved necessary to make a slow but substantial increase in the dosage level. By February 1974 it was up to 5 grams of Brocadopa daily (6 grams during periods of hard work and stress), and inconvenient side-effects were developing. The characteristic 'on/off' or 'swinging' pattern of Parkinson's disease and its treatment had set it, with abrupt and largely unpredictable swings between periods of parkinsonian rigidity and over-active episodes of uncontrollable marionette-like jerkiness.

During September 1976 I changed from levodopa (5.5. grams per day) to Sinemet (1 gram per day), and carefully monitored the effects myself. I had been taking the 22 capsules of Brocadopa one at a time at regular intervals through the waking day. Changing to four Sinemet 275 tablets per day made the intervals between doses too long so I changed to eight half tablets at two-hourly intervals. I also noted that taking Sinemet less than two hours before bed resulted in an over-stimulated and sleepless night. Once the dosage regime was properly adjusted, following discussions with my doctor, the benefits of the reduced levodopa intake became obvious.

By March 1978 the Sinemet dose was raised to 1.5 grams daily, and a home trial of bromocriptine (Parlodel) was started, with a slow reduction in the Sinemet dose. The trial was unsupervised, and I continued to work as usual. Unpleasant and rather frightening symptoms similar to those of shock manifested themselves, and the benefits were at best marginal. Bromocriptine treatment was stopped in July.

In August 1979 treatment with amantadine was

started. This immediately enhanced the beneficial effects of Sinemet, and has continued to do so up to the present time (February 1983). The only unpleasant side-effect I have had from amantadine is occasional heartburn, especially if taken on an empty stomach.

These, then, are the facts of my medical history. But I shall now try to describe the experience of living with the disease and the side-effects of treatment in terms of (a) the symptoms felt by me (b) the outward signs which others see and react to in various ways, and (c) the practical effects on my everyday life and work.

To start with a simple analysis of the pattern: periods of more or less severe muscular rigidity alternate with periods when the muscles are comparatively normal and relaxed; both phases vary in timing and duration (from minutes to hours), but the transition either way is usually abrupt (seconds). These states are totally involuntary; the patient cannot relax by an effort of will. Superimposed on this cycle of rigidity and relaxation are levodopa-induced spells of exaggerated jerky movements (hyperkinesia) alternating with periods of stillness. There is a certain degree of voluntary control over the jerkiness (stillness can be willed, at least briefly), and its severity is much affected by one's emotional state.

Rigidity generally coincides with stillness (the slowness of movement called the hypokinetic parkinsonian state) and relaxation with hyperkinesia, but the two cycles of variation are not always in phase with each other. Hyperkinesia is more irregular in its incidence: rigidity and hyperkinesia can occur together for short periods (the 'paradoxical' state), and so, mercifully, can relaxation and stillness. To confuse matters further, there is an apparent variation in the muscular strength or weakness at different times of day: the pattern is irregular, but seems to be linked with sleepiness or fatigue.

Parkinsonian rigidity is not like the tense rigidity of cramp or arm-wrestling (for example) in normal muscles. It is a dull but constrained inertia, a tight and sluggish unresponsiveness to orders from the brain, and even to unconscious reflexes. It is like trying to swim in treacle – or rather, in jelly, for the parkinsonian 'prison' can tremble violently while remaining implacably closed.

In the rigid state it is extremely difficult to initiate a movement, and equally hard to sustain motion once started. I find that narrow doorways present a peculiar inhibition to taking the first step. Out in the open, however, the hesitating shuffle can, by an act of will, become a long and purposeful stride. It is as though the parkinsonian has two gears, the lower of which is more inhibited. Rhythm, and especially momentum, help movement in the higher 'gear'.

My most serious difficulty at present, and one I find quite unreasonably distressing, is turning over in bed: I can lie down on my back, but (in the rigid phase which usually sets in before bedtime) I have the greatest difficulty turning on to my side. This is a problem of momentum, and one solution is to get out of bed again, pull down the bedclothes, and take a running jump from the far side of the room!

Disturbed balance is another important symptom. There is a real danger of falling over backwards when going upstairs or up a steep hill. Manipulative problems are common in the rigid phase, not only writing but handling papers, knives and forks, clothes, buttons, zips – and going to the lavatory. Extra time has to be allowed for all such tasks and appropriate preparations made during active phases.

The hyperkinetic state, in contrast, is marked by almost uncontrollable fidgeting. The feet shuffle about when seated, and when walking the legs swing in a ludicrously exaggerated manner. A wayward hand, executing a private dance behind one's back, may inadvertently caress a stranger. The eyes are wide and staring, the voice strained and high-pitched. But in general this phase is usually associated with relaxation of the muscles and an escape from the prison of rigidity.

I am left-handed, and from the earliest stages in the progression of the disease it is my left side which has been most affected. My left foot is now persistently turned outward at the ankle and painful to put weight on, so that I walk with a limp. The right foot is normal, except in one respect: if I wake up in the morning still tired after a bad night's sleep, this foot twists inwards in an agonising cramp-like spasm which can affect the whole of the right leg. The cramp is relieved about half an hour after taking the first Sinemet tablet of the day. Baclofen tablets were tried in 1978 for this symptom without success. During the spasm it is impossible to walk on the right foot. I vividly recall standing for nearly an hour on one leg, stork-like, on the pavement outside a book shop in the city of Mainz, while I tried to look up in a pocket dictionary the German words for cramp and ankle.

This brings me to the reactions of other people to parkinsonism. On that occasion in Mainz, the smiling crowds flowed around me as though I were a bollard, and I was glad to be ignored; eventually I caught the eye of an assistant in the shop, who kindly brought me a chair and a cup of tea when I had explained my predicament.

Generally, it is the flamboyant hyperkinetic behaviour which attracts attention on the streets. Girls grin and whisper, small boys laugh and mimic, adults pass by with eyes averted. They presumably think I am drunk, or mad, or both. The rigid state is less ostentatious but evokes a more sympathetic response. I am helped on to buses, offered a seat in shops, and asked if I would like someone to carry purchases to my car.

It is surprising how quickly you learn to ignore, or to become blind to, the unsympathetic reaction to a disability. You grow your own protective shell. It is not so easy for those who love you and are close to you. For that reason I generally go alone, whether I am shopping in the nearby town or travelling to distant places. The family have enough to put up with at home.

I have found my colleagues and my employers very understanding and cooperative. I cannot help feeling ashamed when I measure their continuing loyalty against my declining performance. I particularly appreciate the attitude of the two general practitioners whose patient I have been over the past eighteen years, and of the two specialists who have seen me. They have all treated me as an intelligent and equal partner in an interesting joint enterprise, rather than as a sick man. This is powerful therapy.

Relations and friends have been equally helpful in various ways, taking over responsibilities which I could no longer carry out efficiently, and accommodating sensitively to my changing conditions.

The greatest burden falls inevitably on those whom I love and live with – greater than that on me. My children have had to grow up with a father whose behaviour was more peculiar than that of their friends' fathers, and who was progressively restricted in what he could do for them. They have been marvellous, and as normal as could be; amusing, tolerant and affectionate companions to both their parents.

To my wife I owe my survival. She has had to share with me the struggle to overcome the disability. She has put up with chair arms rubbed threadbare, with clothes stained dark by discoloured sweat, with spilt coffee and food, with amorous advances in the 'window of opportunity' between the seven o'clock Sinemet and time to get up, and with the rarer bouts of hysteria and of near-suicidal depression. She has lost her temper, she has worked herself to exhaustion, she has wept, she has drunk too much, she has cared too much and she has understood. Together we have found that sympathy and softness can do more harm than friendly derision. Every inch of independence must be fought for, and survival depends on facing and mastering new challenges.

Finally some practical effects of the disease. Alcohol in excess, and a high-protein diet (such as steaks) tend to aggravate my parkinsonian rigidity. It is very important to find and stick to the best dosage level and intervals: hospitals please note.

I can still drive a car competently and with enjoyment, provided I take care and avoid the extreme states, of which I get ample forewarning. Apart from changing gear, the mechanical control of a car damps or smooths out minor muscular oscillations and makes driving a comparatively restful activity. Subject to a triennial medical check I am licensed to drive 'a motor car fitted with automatic transmission and vehicles of group A and E with all controls so fitted that they can be correctly and conveniently operated despite intermittent stiffness of left arm and left leg'.

I am taking early retirement at the end of this year. It is a dangerous time, but I look forward to it. There are so many things I want to do. I must learn to fight lassitude and self-pity.

Doctor's comments

To many, this account may give a picture of a man disabled by a particularly severe and complicated form of Parkinson's disease. The author is, in fact, a man of outstanding courage and ability, who has been able to follow a highly successful career in spite of his Parkinson's disease. He has learnt how to overcome many of the problems that the disease and its treatment bring and he has continued in full-time work through eighteen years of the disease. He is above all too modest and too reluctant, to emphasize how successful he has been in leading a normal life at work and at home in spite of his disability. The description he gives makes it clear that the disease can be lived with and solutions to most of the problems can be found. This account should provide inspiration to us all – patients, doctors, friends and family.

Appendix 2

Drugs – Trade Names and Chemical Names

Below are listed the drugs that are used wholly or largely in the treatment of Parkinson's disease. This list includes drugs available on prescription in the United Kingdom and the trade names for the drugs are those used in the United Kingdom.

Trade names are placed in inverted commas. Labelling on a prescribed bottle of tablets or capsules may use either the trade name or the chemical name.

Dopaminergic drugs

Levodopa (L-dopa)

Levodopa capsules	250 mg and 500 mg
Levodopa tablets	500 mg
'Berkdopa' capsules	250 mg and 500 mg clear, marked Berkdopa
'Brocadopa' capsules	125 mg, 250 mg and 500 mg clear capsules
'Brocadopa' tablets	500 mg white, marked with name and strength
'Brocadopa' Temtabs	500 mg
'Larodopa' tablets	500 mg white, marked Roche
'Madopar' (combined levodopa and benserazide) capsules	62.5 blue/grey
	125 blue/pink
	250 blue/caramel
'Sinemet' (combined levodopa and carbidopa) tablets	110 blue, oval, marked MSD 647
	275 blue, oval, marked MSD 654
	plus yellow, marked with tab. name

Amantadine

'Symmetrel' capsules	100 mg dark red, marked in white
'Symmetrel' syrup	50 mg per 5 ml

Bromocriptine

'Parlodel' tablets	2.5 mg white, marked Parlodel
'Parlodel' capsules	10 mg white

Deprenil

'Eldepryl' (selegiline)	5 mg white tablet

Anticholinergic drugs

Benzhexol tablets	2 mg
'Akineton' (biperiden)	2 mg white tablets, marked with a triangle
'Artane' tablets	2 mg and 5 mg white, marked Lederle
Sustets	5 mg turquoise capsule
'Norflex' syrup	5 mg per 5 ml
'Cogentin' (benztropine)	2 mg white tablets MSD 60
'Disipal' (orphenadrine)	50 mg yellow sugar-coated tablets, marked Disipal
'Kemadrin' (procyclidine)	5 mg white, marked Wellcome S3A
'Tremonil' (methixene)	5 mg white tablets, marked Wander

Other drugs mentioned in the text are not listed here because they are not exclusive to Parkinson's disease.

Appendix 3

Useful Names and Addresses

The following information and addresses were supplied by the Parkinson's Disease Society of Great Britain.

Disabled Living Foundation, 346 Kensington High Street, London W14 8NS.
Tel. 01-602 2491.

Parkinson's Disease Society, 36 Portland Place, London W1N 3DG.
(The addresses of local branches can be obtained from head office.)
Tel. 01-323 1174

Royal Association for Disability and Rehabilitation, 25 Mortimer Street, London W1N 8AB.
Tel. 01-637 5400

Local Authority Social Services and Citizens Advice Bureau.
Address available from your local Post Office or public library.

Sexual Problems of the Disabled, 49 Victoria Street, London SW1.

Disablement Income Group, Attlee House, Toynbee Hall, 28 Commercial Street, London E1 6LR.

Scottish Information Service for the Disabled, Claremont House, 18/19 Claremont Crescent, Edinburgh EH7 4QD.
Tel. 031-556 3882

Information Service for Disabled People, Northern Ireland Committee for the Handicapped, 2 Annadole Avenue, Belfast BT7 3JH.
Tel. Belfast 640011

Information Service for the Disabled, Union of Voluntary Organisations for the Handicapped, 29 Eaton Square, Monkstown, Co. Dublin.
Tel. Dublin 809251/803142

Gardens for the Disabled Trust, Headcorn Manor, Headcorn, Kent.

America

American Parkinson Disease Association, 116 John Street, New York, NY 10038.

Parkinson's Disease Foundation, William Black Medical Research Building, 640 West 168th Street, New York, NY 10032.

United Parkinson Foundation, 220 South State Street, Chicago, Illinois 60604.

National Parkinson Foundation, 1501 N.W. 9th Avenue, Miami, Florida 33136.

Parkinson's Educational Program (PEP), 1800 Park Newport, Suite 202–302 Newport Beach, Ca 92660.
Tel. 714/640-0218.

Parkinsonian Society of Greater Washington, 3439 Fourteenth Street North, Arlington, Virginia 22201.

Australia

Mr Don Gration (President), Parkinson's Syndrome Society, 266 Church Street, Parramatta, New South Wales (formed in 1979).

Mrs E. Hemming, Parkinson's Disease Society of Tasmania Inc., 2 Kellatie Road, Montagu Bay, Hobart 7088, Tasmania.

Belgium

Association Pour La Lutte Contre La Maladie de Parkinson, ASBL, Vereniging Voor de Strijd Tegen de Ziekte van Parkinson VZWD, Institut de Medecine, Hospital de Bavière, Bd de la Constitution 66, 4000 Liege.

Canada

Parkinson's Disease Society, 1284 Clyde Avenue, Ottawa, Ontario K2C 1YS.

Parkinson Disease Foundation of Canada, Manulife Centre, Suite 232, 55 Bloor Street West, Toronto, Ontario M4W 1A6.

British Columbia Parkinson's Disease Association, 645 West Broadway, Vancouver, British Columbia V5Z 1G6.

Denmark

Mrs Lisa Hoffmeyer, Immortellevejo 8-2936 Vedback, Denmark.

Eire

Miss M.E. Macaulay, Community and Environment Department, Capel Buildings, 58–71 Great Strand Street, Dublin 1.

Germany

Deutsche Parkinson Vereinigung e.v. Bundesverband, (DPV), Huttenstrasse 7, 4040 Neuss.

Japan

Tokyo Parkinson Patients' Association, Abe Sueo, 3–12 Tsurumki 2–Chome, Setagayaku, Tokyo.

Netherlands

Parkinson Patienten Vereniging Papaver, Prinses Beatrixlaan 5, Bunnik.

New Zealand

Mrs E. Kelly, Field Officer, Southland Parkinson's Disease Society Inc., P.O. Box 1561, Invercargill.

Mr H.M. Schellekena, Parkinson's Disease Society, c/o 148 England Street, Christchurch.

South Africa

The Secretary, South African Parkinsonian Association, CNA Building, 39 Gale Street, Durban, P.O. Box 18151.

Sweden

MS–forbundet, Riksorganisation for neurologiskt, sjuka och handicappade, David Bagares gata 3, 111 38 Stockholm.

Index

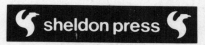